Young People's Experiences of Loss and Bereavement

Young People's Experiences of Loss and Bereavement

Towards an interdisciplinary approach

Jane Ribbens McCarthy

Open University Press

Open University Press
McGraw-Hill Education
McGraw-Hill House
Shoppenhangers Road
Maidenhead
Berkshire
England
SL6 2QL

email: enquiries@openup.co.uk
world wide web: www.openup.co.uk

and Two Penn Plaza, New York, NY 10121–2289, USA

First published 2006

A catalogue record of this book is available from the British Library

ISBN 10: 0335 216 641 (pb) 0335 216 65X (hb)
ISBN 13: 978 0 335 21664 2 (pb) 978 0 335 21665 9 (hb)

Library of Congress Cataloguing-in-Publication Data
CIP data applied for

Typeset by YHT Ltd, London
Printed in Poland by OZGraf S.A.
www.polskabook.pl

To Suzie and Peter

Contents

Tragedy, no one could prepare you, words seem muffled, your chest splits open, the heart skips a million beats then falls slowly but surely to the ground. You try to grab it but it's gone, you're hollow, empty.

You're joking . . . A classic line that's said when faced with such news and of course they're not.

The feeling is like someone pushing hard on your chest, there's air in there but you can't breathe, it's trapped like your state of mind, you're in a thousand places at one time and there's no way out, not now.

So you're on the floor, tears streaming, they roll gently down your cheek until you can taste the salt in the crease of your mouth. It was a grazed knee the last time you tasted it, so much sweeter then.

You're lifted, you're standing, you're stitched up and beating again, then suddenly it all becomes too much and you're back where you started only ten times worse.

Back straight, head hung low, eyes wide and puffy, nose running and lips quivering. You find yourself staring at a plant, it's ugly but you look at it anyway, both hands held, both legs crossed all eyes on you.

You're in shock now, there's no realisation, it can't be true, how could it, things like this don't happen to me I hear you say, but every so often you get a sudden rush of fear, it encloses you with all its power, that's the feeling you get when you believe that this could actually be happening which it is.

Two months, six months, it still comes, that feeling and that tear rolling. Certain things, a smell, a song, a memory, but you grab your heart this time and stick it back in your chest.

No one can prepare you for a tragedy.

Rebecca Willis, aged 15, six months after the death of her stepfather

Before my father died, I thought I knew a bit about bereavement. And I did. A bit. I knew about the shock and the crying; I knew about feeling special, and I had also got a whiff of my own mortality. I knew, intellectually at least, about the anger people are meant to feel when they're bereaved, and in my job as an agony aunt I would blithely send out leaflets to bereaved people – leaflets which told of the stages of grief and were full of kindly, sympathetic advice.

Then my father died. And nothing made sense any more. I was in a new world, with a new language and new emotions. Perhaps he was resting in peace, but I was in utter turmoil. I was stunned, and crazy. Not with grief, but with other shameful feelings of rage, greed, loathing, hatred for life – and with new, surprising interests in religion and the afterlife...

In the same way that a relationship between two people consists of much more than just romantic love (it may not include romantic love at all) and probably includes all kinds of complications – projection, sexual attraction, emotional crutches, trust, neurotic and selfish needs – so there is a great deal more to bereavement than just grief, which is what, of course, makes it so difficult.

Virginia Ironside (1997 p.ix)

Acknowledgements

This project has taken some years to come to fruition and various people have worked on it, in varying capacities, over that time, including (in chronological order): Wendy Martin, Kelvin Street, Julie Jessop, Sue Sharpe, Lynn Eaton and Robert Stephenson. They have all played an important part in diverse ways.

Various individuals and groups have read and commented on draft materials, and some stalwarts have even provided feedback on the whole of an earlier version of the book manuscript. Such commentators have included: Professor Graham Crow, Professor Jenny Hockey, Dr Carol Ann Hooper, Dr Martin Le Voi, Barbara Monroe, Doug Overton, Liz Rolls, Professor Helen Sweeting, the Women's Workshop for Qualitative Household/Family Research and the Centre for Citizenship, Identity and Governance (Open University). Their input has been both encouraging and stimulating, although the author is entirely responsible for any deficiencies in content of the final production.

Professor Janet Holland and Professor Rachel Thompson generously allowed us to develop the case studies in Chapter 3 from data sets held at London South Bank University.

The Joseph Rowntree Foundation and the Open University have provided various elements of funding for the project, and allowed us the time to complete the earlier report (Ribbens McCarthy and Jessop 2005). Special thanks are due to our research manager at the Joseph Rowntree Foundation, Charlie Lloyd, who created the original impetus for the project, and continued to provide patient and interested support.

PART 1
Contexts

1 Knowledge production in context

Introduction

Bereavement is a stage of life evoking even more anxiety than adolescence...
(Walter 1999: 141)

Death and bereavement are issues that contemporary western societies struggle to deal with. Since the period of the Enlightenment, the decline of religion and the march of scientific progress have given rise to a culture which leaves people generally searching to know how to make any sense of death and bereavement, and how to cope with the emotional chaos that may result (Walter 1999). Contemporary western lifestyles increasingly emphasize individual rational choice and self-control, while encounters with death and bereavement may arguably pose challenges to such secularized personal lifestyle projects.

Young people similarly may be seen as threatening to the rational order and self-control of modern civilized society. While the particular anxieties aroused by youth may differ from those aroused by bereavement, from a more general perspective, anthropologists have long pointed out that the boundaries between different social categories or social settings may be fraught with ambiguity and tension. The status of youth, and the status of bereavement, may both be experienced as periods of such marginality, with all the attendant possibilities for uncertainty and disruption.

Both these statuses may also be understood not just as marginal and disruptive, but also as transitional, with youth constituting a time of transition between childhood and adulthood, and bereavement a time of psychosocial transition between one set of significant relationships and another. While the theme of transition does not inevitably connote loss, it does necessarily imply change, and whether or not it is experienced as a loss, change in itself may arouse fears of the unknown and the potentially chaotic. The juxtaposition of bereavement and young people may thus suggest a double jeopardy, invoking deep anxiety, whether among professionals, academics and researchers, or people in their everyday lives, as we consider the transitions and potential disruptions of young people who are experiencing the impact of bereavement.

This book focuses on two particular disparate sets of issues: those concerning the category and experiences of 'young people' on the one hand, and those concerning 'loss' and 'bereavement' on the other,[1] in order to explore what we know about young people's experiences of loss and bereavement in relation to the lives of young people in contemporary western societies, with a particular focus on the UK context. It thus centralizes the question of whether young people do or do not constitute a distinct group in relation to issues relating to bereavement. The purpose of this project has been to consider this question in an open-ended way, identifying and considering what (academic) literatures we have available to us in these areas.

There is now a vast literature, written from the particular cultural contexts of contemporary western societies, that presents theories and research concerning experiences and implications of (major) bereavement. The potential for emotional chaos after bereavement may, however, defy such attempts to develop a sense of theoretical or empirical coherence and orderliness (as Ironside 1997 eloquently argues – see p. ix). And indeed, Walter (1999) suggests that bereavement may at times share some of the characteristics of mental disorder. Thus Craib (1994), in discussing C.S. Lewis's profound autobiographical account of the disorderly experience of bereavement, argues that grief is a (potentially never-ending) process or history, *not* a state about which a map can be drawn. There is also a vast but largely separate literature that seeks to develop an orderly understanding of the position and development of young people, but the experiences of adolescence and youth may similarly refuse to fall into the neat lines set by such endeavours.

Furthermore, our[2] approach has also involved keeping open the question of when a 'significant' bereavement experience may imply a major disruption in a young person's biography – with the potential for upheaval in both the short- and long-term – and when bereavement may carry fewer implications for the individual's life course overall but may nevertheless constitute an important aspect of a young person's experience. The existing bereavement literature focuses much more strongly on 'significant' bereavements than it does on young people's experiences of bereavement in more general terms.

In undertaking a review of some of the relevant literatures, this project provides the opportunity to develop an overview, or map, of the ways in

---

[1] We discuss the meaning of our key terms in Chapter 2, and see Ribbens McCarthy and Jessop (2005) for an account of how we conducted the literature search.

[2] The 'we' in this discussion at times refers to all three of the individuals who have been directly employed on this project at some point, including Julie Jessop, Wendy Martin and Jane Ribbens McCarthy. However, not all of this discussion necessarily reflects the views of all of us as individuals. At other points, it refers to all those who are working or writing in these areas. Sue Sharpe's contribution to the project was undertaken in a consultancy capacity. See Acknowledgements for a list of people who have contributed over time.

which 'lay' accounts, academic work, policies and professional interventions have produced particular views and frameworks regarding these two sets of issues. In the process, there may perhaps be scope for asking questions about how and why theories and associated empirical findings are formulated in the ways that they are at present – why the contours of this 'map' occur as they do, why the frontiers are placed where they are, whether there are further uncharted areas for exploration, and how far these features have arisen from the social processes of knowledge production, rather than constituting fixed and inevitable features of the landscape. We cannot claim to have produced fully exhaustive reviews of all the various areas of research we discuss. However, although we may not have uncovered every relevant publication, we have looked at a great array of materials, arguably enough to have built quite a solid picture of the findings and evidence.

But these questions are not just a matter of detached academic curiosity – the focus on the pressing substantive issue of young people's experiences of bereavement points to the urgent need to develop an interdisciplinary dialogue based on a constructive engagement between different perspectives and different professions. At the same time, our focus here raises much broader issues about the social production of knowledge, and the possibilities for changing some of the contours of the existing maps – through a dialogue across current disciplinary and methodological boundaries.

In exploring these literatures we sought not to foreclose any of these issues, but instead to reflect on the underlying assumptions of the ways in which their contours are currently drawn. In some respects, then, we are here setting out on a major journey, through all sorts of different landscapes, and with only fragments of a map to guide us. We have therefore had to find our own pathway through these issues, seeking to avoid any artificial or premature imposition of order, while at the same time recognizing the need to develop signposts that provide some sense of orientation.

In this process, we have found ourselves straying beyond the general borderlands of academic thinking as this is framed by the modernist projects of rational thought and empirically-based control. As Virginia Ironside hints (see p. ix), close encounters with these topics inevitably raise questions about our own mortality and search for meaning in life, as well as how we can respond to, and make sense of, some of the most profound issues of human relationships, of our deepest attachments, security and suffering.

The threat to meaning, indeed to any sense of what is 'real', is only too graphically apparent in Rebecca Willis's portrayal of the shock of the death of someone dearly loved (see p. viii). Not only may bereaved young people find themselves considering such dilemmas of loss and meaning, but so too do writers of the academic literatures we will be exploring in this book, whether or not they themselves explicitly discuss this. Perhaps inevitably, undertaking this work has also, in the end, required us to reflect explicitly on our own spiritual or existential understandings, and their relevance to our academic work and writing in the course of this project.

How we attribute 'meaning' to bereavement, whether in general terms or by reference to the death of a particular individual, is thus a central theme of this book on many different levels. It is explored firstly in this Chapter as we reflect on the processes of (scientific) knowledge production that underpin our current understandings of young people and bereavement, and consider how subjective and existential dilemmas of meaning may or may not be addressed by such knowledge. It is then discussed in relation to the broad cultural contexts of death and dying in western societies at this point in history – cultural contexts which give rise to particular meanings that are incorporated into the theoretical perspectives we have available to us in relation to young people and bereavement (Chapter 2). Having thus considered some of the broader contexts and issues that underpin our knowledge in Part 1, we then turn in Part 2 to examine the existing research evidence more closely. We begin by considering issues of meaning in the context of individual lives, through the qualitative research evidence, and in particular presenting new case studies of five young people who have very variable experiences of bereavement (Chapter 3). Subsequent chapters then present the existing published research evidence, covering issues of bereavement as a statistically defined 'risk' factor in the individual life trajectory (Chapter 4), and the implications for social relationships, informal social contexts, and the institutionalized settings of schools and specialist bereavement organizations (Chapter 5), before returning in Part 3 to a discussion of how far an emphasis on 'meaning' might usefully provide a basis for greater interdisciplinarity and multi-methods approaches (Chapter 6). In the process, the meaning of 'meaning' is itself explored, particularly in the contexts of human suffering, mortality, and the urge to survive and thrive in the various challenges and experiences of life.

A hidden issue?

Young people are generally understood to be in the process of leaving the innocence of childhood behind, an innocence that is underpinned by a measure of protection from some of the harsher realities of life. One such reality is that of death, and the implications that ensue from bereavement. We may have come to expect children to be protected from this experience, particularly in affluent western societies where average life expectancy has extended dramatically over the last century. As a result of this major demographic shift, which is underpinned by the affluence of western industrialized economies, we may often expect children to have little direct contact with death among those nearest to them, at least for a major part of their childhood.

Material affluence may also be seen to underpin the establishment of childhood itself, as a distinct phase of the life course, in the particular social and historical circumstances of western industrialized societies. While childhood may seem to be rooted in the 'natural' processes of physical and mental immaturity, the 'new' childhood studies of recent decades have drawn our attention to the ways in which the historical development of particular, institutionally and legally based, frameworks for the lives of the younger members of society, has led to a specific view of childhood as a protected time of innocence that in many respects should be lived out, and kept apart from, some of the more difficult or risky experiences of adult lives (see e.g. Ennew 1986; Ribbens 1994; James *et al.* 1998; Alanen and Mayall 2001; Maybin and Woodhead 2003).

Young people are thus commonly understood to be facing a major life 'transition', as they move from the status of Child to that of Adult,[3] a process entailing numerous changes in the context of contemporary industrialized societies. Such life changes have become increasingly ambiguous and uneven in many ways in recent decades, as various writers have discussed (Alanen and Mayall 2001; Jones 2002). On the one hand, childhood may be described as having been eroded, particularly through an exposure to mass media, but on the other hand adulthood may be said to have receded, as participation in the education system has been prolonged and financial and residential independence have become harder to achieve (Brannen *et al.* 2002; Jones 2005).

In other ways, however, it may also be argued that childhood has become even more idealized and institutionalized, particularly via marketing and consumption related to family events such as Christmas, and special sites such as Disneyland. The status of Child in western societies has shifted from that of potential economic asset to an economic liability that is undertaken regardless, as children are perceived as priceless, forming the centre of adult hopes and desires for an enduring bond in the face of modern uncertainties (Zelizer 1994). At the same time, the status of Adult may be seen to carry ever more arduous burdens for self-responsibility, as individuals make their

---

[3] The use of the capitals for Child and Adult is intended to signal that we are not talking here directly about actual children and adults, but about the positions or socially constructed statuses that particular individuals are expected to occupy by virtue of chronological criteria. Actual individuals may at times place themselves, or be placed by others, in one or other of these categories regardless of their chronology (e.g. see Ribbens McCarthy and Edwards 2000). Such challenges to the generally fixed linkage between chronological age and generational status may be experienced by people as very disturbing. This may be exemplified by children who are said to have had their childhood cut short by being burdened too young by Adult responsibilities or knowledge, as with children caring for disabled adults, or child sexual abuse.

choices in a consumerist society, and chart their individual, reflexive bio-graphies to shape their own destinies (Giddens 1991, 1992).

There has been considerable attention paid in recent years to the various ways in which young people and their families may deal with these difficult, often unexpected, and arguably increasingly complex, processes of change. Within these discussions, however, one significant possible source of life change has been neglected, namely experiences of death and bereavement that may add to the complexities of the disruptions and transitions of the teenage and early adult years.

On the one hand, death and bereavement are topics that contemporary western societies may struggle to make sense of, preferring to leave the ma-terial realities of human mortality to specialist sites and services (see Chapter 2). Perhaps related to this unease about the outer limits of the rational pro-gress of modernity, adults may seek to protect children from knowledge of adult inability – despite all the baffling wonders of technological advances – to shape and protect life from pain, death and loss. On the other hand, concerns and anxieties regarding the lives of young people that surface in academic and policy debates have tended to focus on broad issues that may be expected to relate to the category of youth *en masse*, or to issues of the control of particularly troublesome, deviant individuals. Bereavement has thus re-ceived little attention within broader debates concerned with the lives of young people.

The social context of this book

While seeking to develop a map of relevant knowledge to further our un-derstanding of this area of experience, part of the picture must also include a consideration of how this book itself features within this landscape. Our writing here originates from a project funded by the Joseph Rowntree Foun-dation, who had decided that this topic was ripe for more specific attention than it had received to date. This raises the question of why this focus seems to have become especially pertinent at this time. As we attended conferences and networks, and made contact with active professional organizations in the course of the project, it became apparent that other bodies had also been asking questions about this specific area of potential need. We can speculate about the possible reasons for this, which may comprise a number of fairly disparate threads.

On the one hand, the hospice movement in Britain has expanded apace in recent decades, and continues to do so, in the face of rising cancer rates particularly. The hospice movement comprises numerous and varied local initiatives and activities, generally seen by those involved to be meeting a desperate need for new ways of caring for people who are terminally ill. As hospices have become more established and the needs of terminally ill people have become more widely recognized, new needs have become apparent, in relation to those close to the dying person – family members and friends who may be involved in their care and who will experience the death as a significant and traumatic loss. Hospices have thus increasingly extended their remit to incorporate services for those who are bereaved by the death, and the remit of palliative care has broadened constantly. This has then, in turn, opened up new areas of perceived need, namely those of children who are bereaved, leading on to the further consideration of how and whether the needs of young people need separate consideration from those of children generally.[4]

In a different direction altogether, bereavement may have come to the attention of policy-makers concerned with sources of social exclusion in relation to the lives of young people. A few of the studies which have focused on such issues have pointed to some unexpected findings about the possible relevance of bereavement in the life histories of particularly vulnerable or deviant young people, particularly where research has used biographical approaches to understand how life processes may occur over time (e.g. Johnston *et al.* 2000; Barry 2001). More broadly, some of the ways in which processes of change during the teenage years are seen to be currently changing may have led, as Wyn and White (1997) suggest, to an (uneven) shift of emphasis away from a view of young people as problematic, to one of young people as victims, a view with which bereavement issues would be consonant.

These two strands of activity – development of specialist services for young people within the voluntary sector for the dying and bereaved, and biographical studies of vulnerable young people that have pointed to bereavement issues – may together have led to the question at the centre of this project: what do we know about young people's experiences of bereavement? This is a topic that *potentially* invokes, and links with, a wide variety of existing debates and literatures, depending on how the question is theorized.

The key concepts of this project – young people, bereavement and loss – point to further questions about how far bereavement may be seen as a source of change or loss equivalent to other changes or disruptions in the lives and relationships of young people. What is particularly striking, when viewed in this broader context of debate about family disruptions, is that bereavement potentially casts the bereaved as 'victims of circumstance', without the

---

[4] As this process continues, it seems that additional needs may become a focus for concern, as hospices become aware of other categories of grieving people, such as those who have been bereaved by sudden or traumatic deaths without any previous contact with services for dying and bereaved people, but who contact organizations in their search for services that may help bereaved adults, children or young people.

potential for stigma that is apparent in relation to other forms of family disruption. We are hardly likely to see a moral panic arising about widowed mothers as presiding over deviant forms of household in the way that we have seen moral panics arising regarding divorced, separated or single teenage mothers (Duncan and Edwards 1999). At the same time, it has to be recognized that bereavement does not pose the same thorny issues for legislation that are posed by divorce, which may have contributed to its invisibility as a topic for policy-makers.

If we consider bereavement in the context of other forms of family change and disruption, it is possible that what can be learned in the context of bereaved families may have the potential to shed light on alternative ways of approaching other forms of family disruption, particularly in terms of policies or practices that might be found to be supportive without being felt to be stigmatizing. Nevertheless, we also have to recognize that any form of difference, that others find difficult to deal with, may be felt in some ways as a source of stigma. There is evidence, for example (discussed in Chapter 5), that bereaved children may find the loss of a parent through death can be used as a basis for bullying or name-calling in ways similar to other forms of difference.

The social contexts of (cross-disciplinary) knowledge production

In asking how the focus of this project has crystallized from various ongoing social organizations and policy debates, and considering what light may be shed on the topic from existing academic literatures, we are also raising questions about the social contexts and processes underlying the production of academic knowledge. Some aspects of the contours of the maps we will draw in this book are the outcomes of complex interweaving processes that lead to a layered and mutually influential interconnection between individual personal experiences, professional activities, academic debates and ongoing collective activities in localized contexts. Furthermore, these processes may be viewed from a broader sociohistorical framework (see Chapter 2), as part of a search to find some sense of meaning, and to develop appropriate social practices, that can help us live with the awesome significance of death and bereavement in a largely secular society. Such an approach could – but need not necessarily – be framed by reference to a Foucauldian analysis of knowledge/power in relation to the complex ways in which 'knowledge' is 'produced' and becomes interwoven with professional and personal discourses and practices, such that it becomes part of an implicit internal 'surveillance' (see Walter 1999; Small and Hockey 2001).

In such processes, individual experiences of bereavement may lead people to come together in organized endeavours to meet perceived individual needs, which are then developed in conjunction with professional and voluntary sector perspectives, along with 'expert' theorizing that may arise out of, and feed into, these localized experiences and perspectives. One particularly significant aspect of this process, perhaps, concerns the relationship between research and professional and lay practices. The 'expert' theories that have developed out of these various contexts may become incorporated into everyday 'common sense' or 'lay' understandings of bereavement, which are then taken to validate the underlying perspectives: 'The negotiation of normality between experts, popular culture and bereaved individuals is an ongoing feature of the social world of bereavement' (Walter 1999: 165). In this sense we may draw a broad parallel with Giddens's discussion of the reflexive nature of sociology, in that all academic knowledge develops within particular social contexts that are not hermetically sealed from ongoing social processes, but *inter*relate with people's everyday understandings, and organizational agendas, in complex and subtle ways.

Importantly, then, such social contexts provide variable frameworks for the validation of knowledge about young people and bereavement. Particular audiences may receive such knowledge in relation to various academic, professional or personal frames of relevance, which shape the issues that people want such knowledge to address, the purposes they hope it will fulfil and the nature of the evidence by which they will be convinced.

Disciplinary perspectives and methodological divergences

Each of the potentially relevant literatures, based in different disciplines and associated differences of empirical evidence, invokes and depends upon variable epistemological underpinnings and methodological strategies. There may thus be differences regarding each literature's choice of concepts, definition of key questions, and ideas about what sort of research methods are appropriate in providing evidence that is accepted as valid within the terms of reference of that discipline and methodology. In this sense, each area of academic knowledge may carry different implicit meanings in the ways in which issues of death and bereavement are framed.

In exploring and discussing these different aspects of the literature, then, we see it as entirely appropriate to shift our own epistemological position in different discussions, rather than taking a single stance on what sorts of evidence are considered to be relevant and valid. Some evidence, for example, depends on longitudinal quantitative data that are subjected to highly sophisticated statistical manipulation in order to 'test' for 'causal' links and processes; some depends on clinical experience and 'case histories'; while other evidence again may depend upon an exploration and detailed examination of the 'discourses' or 'narratives' by which individual young people 'make sense' of their life experiences over time. Each of these approaches has a part to play, and we would not want here necessarily to accord priority to any one in particular, rather seeking to consider the underlying frameworks of each, while also paying careful attention to the conclusions reached within those parameters, and the possibilities for dialogue between them.

But in recognizing the social processes and contexts underlying the various writings on bereavement and young people, we have also been conscious of our own biographies, experiences and understandings that have shaped, and continue to shape, our particular interests and perspectives in this area. As individuals working on this project, we brought varied direct experiences of bereavement, both personally and professionally, including parents, partners, friends and the children of friends, and sometimes with young children or young people being directly bereaved themselves. We also brought a variety of academic and professional perspectives to this work – including family sociology, medical sociology, palliative care nursing, and work in national policy and pressure groups of varying types. While seeking an interdisciplinary dialogue, then, it is also important to recognize that its starting point in this book is rooted in our own primary backgrounds in sociology.

'Meaning' and 'suffering'

Reflecting on the relevance of our own biographies, however, has also led us to questions about the biographies and experiences of all of those who feel able, and want, to work in such a difficult area of interest. As others have argued (e.g. Masson and Gieve 2003), even the most supposedly detached of professional individuals, such as judges and doctors, may find that working in these areas raises deep pain and fears of death and suffering, whether recognized or not. While we have had to struggle with, and manage, the boundaries between our own personal experiences and this public, academic project, we have been led to wonder about the coping responses of others in this field. It seems clear that not everyone feels comfortable with work that focuses on bereavement and loss, so are the people who do work in and write about this subject quite a particular, self-selected set of individuals? Is the academic literature produced by people who find it helpful to look directly at these issues, rather than those who prefer not to think too directly about such difficult aspects of our lives? And if this speculation has some relevance, what are the consequences for the literature that is produced?

Some authors and practitioners suggest that these topics can only be fully addressed by recognizing and embracing their spiritual implications, whether these are framed by institutionalized religion or more broadly as 'a desire to find purpose and fulfilment ... a search for meaning, faith and hope, and a recognition of the wholeness and value of life' (Gordon 2001: 84). In this respect, 'meaning' may be understood in terms of 'purpose', but others may prefer not to define such issues through this language of purposefulness and spirituality, perhaps thinking instead in terms of existential or philosophical debates. Thompson, for example, suggests that the primary focus of all social work is to help people deal with 'existential challenges' (2002: 13), in terms of the demands we experience as human beings. Moss (2002: 35) suggests that 'It is, perhaps, in our experiences of loss, especially significant loss, that we face most acutely the whole question of meaning'. From this perspective, loss may be experienced as a crisis precisely because it may also entail a loss of meaning. Others again define spirituality itself – which is seen to be 'fundamental to the human person' – primarily as a 'quest for meaning' (Morgan 2002: 195).

Others again might prefer not to think at all about such issues that appear to lie outside the realms of rational thought and/or (what some would regard as) empirically based certainties and knowledge. Moss (2002) argues that, nevertheless, questions of meaning are unavoidable, both for individuals and professionals facing situations of significant loss. To refuse to perceive such questions as relevant, Moss argues, amounts to a 'flight from self-awareness'. And, as we shall see in subsequent chapters, even the most scientific of approaches may find themselves having to take 'meanings' into account, with regard to the subjective interpretations that people themselves place upon events.

In a broader discussion, Morgan and Wilkinson (2001: 211) have argued that the social sciences have appeared indifferent to such issues precisely because of the deep tensions between modernity's expectations of moral progress (see Chapter 2), and the realities of exploitation and suffering in the modern world. They call for work towards a new 'sociodicy' which will help forefront, analyse and critique this tension, work which incorporates the need to document suffering in people's lives:

> We suggest that all forms of suffering, whether emotional or physical, individual or collective, are liable to raise fundamental questions about the significance and purpose of life. Although physical pain may be distinguished from existential angst, and genocide from an isolated instance of torture or rape, in all such cases, the sheer irrationality of suffering confronts us with an unbearable absence of moral reasoning.

We return in more detail to questions of 'meaning' in Chapter 6. But as we undertake our overview of the literatures in the intervening chapters, it is important to bear in mind that such spiritual, existential or philosophical issues may underlie the varying (often very heated and apparently deeply felt) debates that we shall encounter. Debates that consider, for example, whether young people bereaved of a parent are at substantially increased risk of depression, or how best we can respond to the pain and confusion of bereaved young people, as well as how we can assess the depth and extent of such pain. What has been apparent to us, as readers new to these literatures and debates, is that there is an enormous energy and commitment from people devoted to helping alleviate such pain, while there are also others who seem equally committed to the argument that such pain is really not so bad or so extensive, and that some interventions may be quite misplaced.[5] Furthermore, such debates raise implications, not only for the commitment of individuals, but also for the commitment of public resources, for example, through the provision of medical or educational services (Small 2001a). At times these concerns seem to have led writers to a rather haphazard, selective, and on occasions completely inappropriate citing of sources to try to convince others of the validity of particular viewpoints. We have thus been very concerned to find not just one, but several, writers who appear to rely on sources that are either entirely irrelevant, or even directly contradictory, to the arguments for which they are being cited in support.

In considering why people (including ourselves) want to work in this area, we have considered various philosophical, emotional and spiritual stances that may underlie the apparently detached 'scientific' or 'professional' writings and work. Is it that we want to put things 'right' for suffering individuals, as the pain or confusion seems so unbearable we are impelled to the belief that it *can* be put right? Is it that we want to believe that we can at least find some sort of (purposeful) meaning in the midst of pain, so that it does not amount to just pointless suffering? Is it that we want to assure ourselves that things are not *really* so bad? Those of a psychoanalytic leaning might well perceive all sorts of psychic defence mechanisms at play in the context of such issues, including denials and projections (Craib 1994) (and we return in Chapter 2 to issues of contemporary social contexts for emotional responses to bereavement).

What is very clear is that the vast majority of what has been written about these areas is oriented towards the issue of interventions: about *how* we can or should help; or how it is *not necessary* to help because we have overestimated the suffering involved and its consequences; or how it is possible to find some sense of purpose or *meaning*, such as personal growth, through the intense pain and confusion that may accompany bereavement. In considering such issues with regard to our own motivations, we have been reminded of what is known as 'the serenity prayer' (the insight and relevance of which does not

---

[5] Hockey (1990) offers an unusually open reflection on this impelling need to feel able to help those who seem overwhelmed by pain, when she discusses her experiences as a bereavement counsellor undertaking an ethnography of dying and bereavement.

depend on any particular belief about God), which is widely used in various support groups for problematic life experiences:

> God grant me the serenity to accept the things I cannot change
> Courage to change the things I can
> And wisdom to know the difference.

Although we are tempted (very presumptiously) to add an additional prayer, to help us to know what, or whether, anything needs to be changed in the first place. Perhaps it is relevant to bear in mind the words of the first (fourteenth-century) woman writer in English, Julian of Norwich: '... suffering is transient ... but all shall be well, and all shall be well, and all manner of things shall be well (1998: 50–1).

Continuities and differences

While the spiritual or existential dilemmas raised by experiences of death and bereavement in the lives of young people may be inescapable, it is also imperative that we recognize that not all bereavement experiences necessarily entail suffering – although we would argue that they always point to questions of meaning (see Chapter 6). Indeed, as mentioned above, bereavement may also be understood in a more open-ended way as a source of change, and indeed, not necessarily as a form of loss (a point we will consider further in Chapter 2).

At the level of the experiences of young people themselves, then, we may distinguish between:

- death and bereavement as 'normal' experiences in the lives of young people;
- bereavement that has significance for major emotional or biographical disruption, raising issues, perhaps, of increased vulnerability, identity and a sense of difference or stigma.

There may be a parallel here with other issues (e.g. see Newburn and Shiner's 2001 discussion of the significance of alcohol consumption) in the lives of young people, during their years of transition, as they leave the (idealized) 'protection' of childhood behind. Are death and bereavement an aspect of 'growing up' that all young people have to deal with, a 'normal' part of the teenage learning curve, while for some particular young people it may become a dominating and highly disruptive feature of their lives?

Given the major historical decline in early mortality since the nineteenth century (Anderson 1990), and the absence of wars involving large numbers of young people from western countries over the last 60 years, we might expect that children and young people generally are unlikely to have direct experience of bereavement, but this is not the case. While the existing evidence is not clear about the frequency of experience of particular categories of death (see Ribbens McCarthy and Jessop 2005), overall, the great majority (as high as 92 per cent) of young people in the UK do report having experienced bereavement with regard to what they consider to be a 'close' or 'significant' relationship (sometimes including pets), before the age of 16 (Harrison and Harrington 2001). Such experiences will be even more common by the age of 18 or 25. Evidence from the USA suggests similarly high levels. Ewalt and Perkins (1979) for example, found that 90 per cent of high-school students reported having seen a dead person and had lost someone they cared about.

While many of these bereavements concern the death of a grandparent, or other second-degree relative, the death of a parent before age 16 is not as uncommon as might be supposed. Figures in the UK range from 3.9 per cent (Sweeting *et al.* 1998) to 7.4 per cent (Wadsworth 1991), while in the USA figures range from 5 per cent (Kliman 1979 cited by Gersten *et al.* 1991; Wessel 1983 cited by Servaty and Hayslip 2001) to 11 per cent (Ewalt and Perkins 1979). Ayers *et al.* (2003) cite data from the US Social Security Administration showing that 6.1 per cent of adolescents between the ages of 13 and 17 had experienced the death of a parent (a figure that will, of course, rise by the time all these young people reach 18).

Figures for the death of a sibling are harder to establish, but seem to be similar to (or perhaps slightly lower than) figures for the death of a parent (Harrison and Harrington 2001). The majority of sibling deaths will concern the death of an infant. The prevalence of bereavement due to the death of a close friend is yet more elusive to establish, but there is some evidence to suggest that this may be two or three times more common than these 'family' deaths. Meltzer *et al.* (2000) found twice as many 5–15-year-olds in the UK reported the death of a close friend as the death of a parent or sibling, and Harrison and Harrington (2001) estimated that 16 per cent of young people would experience the death of a close friend by age 16, while Ewalt and Perkins (1979) found that 40 per cent of high-school students in one locality in Kansas had experienced the death of a close friend their own age. Balk and McNeil (1990 cited by Balk 1991b) found that over 30 per cent of a sample of college undergraduates reported that a close friend had died within the preceding 12 months, and over 45 per cent said that a close friend had died within the past two years. Among young people in the USA, especially, violent deaths may be particularly significant, with a rise in mortality rates apparent among 15–24-year-old males between 1960 and 1980 (Berman 1986 cited by Balk 1995). While this pattern has not been apparent in the UK, mortality rates for this age group do nevertheless continue to be much higher than for younger males (Charlton 1996).

The likelihood of young people experiencing bereavements will also vary by locality and across particular social circumstances. We know, for example, that life expectancy varies very significantly by social class, geography and locality, and such health inequalities have widened in the UK in recent years (Shaw 1999; Mitchell *et al.* 2000). The risk of premature death (i.e. before aged 65) is almost three times greater in some parliamentary constituencies than others, and the risk of death is further related to living in deprived localities. So we would expect the experience of bereavement due to death of a parent to vary significantly by social class and locality too, with young people living in deprived areas being more likely to experience the death of a parent. Death of a sibling is likely to vary in similar ways, with infant mortality, for example, being strongly related to the father's social class (Schuman 1998): 'In Britain as a whole over one quarter of childhood deaths . . . were attributable to social inequality' (Shaw 1999: 162).

Variations in mortality rate according to ethnic group are not so well established in the UK, partly because ethnic group is not recorded on death certificates, so that studies can only instead undertake analyses by the country of origin of immigrants. Standardized all-cause mortality rates are only slightly higher among men and women born in the Indian sub-continent and women born in the Caribbean compared with the general population, while they are slightly lower among men born in the Caribbean (Nazroo 2001). This contrasts quite markedly with the higher mortality rates among those born in Ireland or Scotland and living in England and Wales (Wild and Mckeigue 1997). Nevertheless, the breakdown of the figures shows the importance of looking at specific sub-groups. Bangladeshi-born men, for example, have been found to have significantly higher mortality rates than those for the general population for England and Wales (Balarajan and Soni Raleigh 1997). At a theoretical as well as an empirical level, Nazroo (2001) argues that an analysis of variations in mortality and health between ethnic groups requires careful attention to issues of socioeconomic class, as well as racial identity and experiences of racism. In the USA, however, one study that specifically considered ethnicity as a factor in the bereavement experiences of a nationally representative sample of teenagers, found that ethnicity as well as household income was related to the likelihood of experiencing the death of a friend (Rheingold et al 2004).

Overall, then, it is clear that the vast majority of young people – whatever their circumstances – experience the death of a close or significant person in their lives before the age of 18. In this sense, bereavement is a statistically 'normal' part of growing up. On the other hand, death of a member of the immediate family – particularly a parent or sibling – may be more of a minority experience, albeit a fairly substantial minority, particularly for some localities and social groups.

How we trace such continuities and discontinuities of experiences has major implications for any interventions we may see as appropriate. There is thus a major tension between specialist approaches and broader lay and public discourses regarding death and bereavement. This is paralleled in many ways by a tension between specialist and generic services, whether the specialism is focused on bereavement as a particular experience, or youth as a particular category of people. What is readily apparent, however, is that the existing academic and research literature overwhelmingly focuses on experiences of difference and disruption in relation to bereavement, and we know very little about issues of death and bereavement in the lives of young people generally. We have very little evidence to know whether bereavement might be understood, for example, within the general context of the life course as entailing all sorts of disruptions over the years, or whether it is indeed viewed as a disruption of a *different kind*. These themes of 'difference' and 'continuity' will constitute an overarching theme for the discussion in subsequent chapters. Is it helpful that literature and expertise on this topic are at present quite so clearly demarcated and specialized, or is there scope for identifying links and continuities with other features of the lives of young people? Again, we will return to such issues in Chapter 6.

Conclusions

At the start of this project, we were aware that we ourselves were each in different ways entering new academic terrain. What has been exciting both academically and personally, however, has been to find the ways in which this terrain is not necessarily new to us at all, but can be found to have all sorts of continuities with other areas of academic work. It is this subjective experience that we have used to focus a central theme of this project, concerning how far the topic of young people and bereavement can be found to have continuities with other experiences and bodies of work, and how far it is found to be a distinctly 'different' area of work, the province of specialist expertise. Where are boundaries and differences found, and where continuities, and why?

In undertaking the literature search, what became apparent quite quickly is that there is a specialist literature available (although sometimes embedded in other work) if the topic is defined in a clearly bounded way (see Chapter 2). To have drawn such tight boundaries would have lightened our task in reviewing the literature, but would itself have contributed to a further reinforcement of such boundaries, and a closing down, perhaps, of potential links and debates. But if we want to treat such boundaries as contingent, and reflect upon the ways in which the boundaries are drawn, we find that the more specialised materials implicate a vast array of academic and professional literatures, as well as many different areas of social policy and practice.

In mapping these various literatures, then, we have drawn the contours by reference to certain features of the landscape that are not necessarily immutable, being the result of the particular social contexts in which the academic literatures are embedded. We therefore hope that, by making these contours more explicit from the perspective of this particular overview, it may be possible to see how the map could be drawn differently, if more connections were made – perhaps enabling new synergies – or different vantage points were adopted.

We have struggled not to be overwhelmed by these potentials, and have not attempted here to develop such links. Indeed, our approach has meant that we consider many complex issues with some brevity. Nevertheless, we hope our endeavours will provide a fruitful contribution towards consolidating some of the existing work, and pointing to further potential. In the process we have found that our specific substantive focus leads towards major issues of social theory and interdisciplinarity which may themselves be fruitfully considered by reference to the light they may or may not be able to shed on the issues at stake.

2 Young people, death and bereavement in contemporary western societies[1]

Introduction

In this chapter, we will attempt to provide an overview of the theoretical discussions that underpin the academic and other literatures that are concerned with bereavement and young people. We will start with a consideration of how the social and personal position of young people may be theorized, and the implications of this for understanding young people's experiences of bereavement. We will then discuss the broad sociohistorical theorizing of death and dying, before turning to the more psychological concepts of bereavement and grief, and their theoretical associations. This consideration of the theorizing of youth and bereavement, and of the contexts in which such theories have themselves developed, is an essential precursor to any understanding of how the specific literature on bereavement and young people has been framed, and how it is underpinned by certain assumptions.

The contours of 'young people' as a category and a literature

One of the first questions people often asked when we said we were doing this work was, what did we mean by 'young people'? Initially we sought to keep open the theoretical space for how we might think about this age group, defining our area of interest by a loose reference to the teenage years and the early twenties. However, even this approach of course carries theoretical implications of the potential significance of age.

There are two major approaches to theorizing the teenage years that can be found in the academic literature, and both seep through to the

---

[1] We wish to acknowledge the particular input of earlier working papers written by Wendy Martin that underpin some sections of this chapter.

professional and self-help literatures on bereavement, though not to an equal degree. The two approaches can be broadly identified as:

- A view of the teenage years as indicating the period of 'adolescence', which is rooted very strongly in the psychological literatures, and often connotes a view of the teenage years as shaped by biological changes (discussed further below), sometimes characterized as 'storm and stress' (Gillies 2001).
- A view of the teenage years as indicating the institutionally-based status of being a 'young person' or part of a category of 'youth': 'youth' is a specific process in which young people engage with institutions such as schools, the family, the police, welfare and many others' (Wyn and White 1997: 3).

This approach is rooted very strongly in the sociological and social policy literature, and often connotes a view of the teenage years as a time of 'transition' between the statuses of childhood and adulthood (as discussed in Chapter 1).

The implications of these divergent theoretical frameworks have been explored, for example, in relation to the family lives of young people (Gillies 2001), but there has not been any equivalent consideration in relation to bereavement issues. Instead, in line with the generally psychological underpinnings of the bereavement literature, the theoretical framework of 'adolescence' is heavily predominant. There is ambiguity sometimes in this approach about the ways in which adolescence may be defined by reference to physical/biological changes and/or by reference to chronological age. Balk (1995), for example, identifies three periods of adolescence chronologically, although later he suggests that it is puberty that marks the beginning of adolescence:

- early adolescence, 10–14 years;
- middle adolescence, 15–17 years;
- late adolescence, 18–22 years.

Some writers within the general theoretical perspective of adolescence do nevertheless indicate some consideration of its potential basis in social contexts. Corr and McNeil, for example, write that 'adolescence is the product of a certain set of circumstances (among which is increased life expectancy) wherein society acknowledges a kind of interval between childhood and young adulthood' (1986: xii).

The writings of Balk are particularly relevant here, as he writes both in general terms about adolescent development, and (unusually) also pays particular attention to issues of bereavement. Balk argues that the word 'adolescence' is not new, having been part of (presumably Anglo-Saxon) language for several centuries. In his theoretical framework, drawing on the work of Erikson, identity formation is seen as a central developmental task, such that 'A key developmental task for adolescents is to separate from parents and to live independently as a young adult' (Balk 1995: 272). This is contextualized, however, by a discussion as to whether ideas about identity formation in adolescence are 'the product of an Anglo-American culture that prizes independence and individuation over communal investment and fidelity to traditions' (1995: 140). Balk also discusses evidence that working-class youths (implicitly male?) may develop their identities differently from college students, but it is the latter that have been used to develop much of the research on identity formation.

Nevertheless, while these issues are discussed at specific points in Balk's work, most of the different areas of life course change are theorized and discussed as stages that are universal and invariant. Similarly, Hogan and DeSantis (1994) suggest that there is likely to be a worldwide increase in the numbers of adolescents experiencing sibling bereavement, without discussing the very different social and cultural contexts for such a phenomenon – such as social violence, AIDS, suicides, civil and international conflict – and the significance of such contexts for the experience of sibling bereavement. They discuss the ways in which research should aim to identify 'normal' processes of adolescent sibling bereavement, and what helps to lead to resilience or vulnerability, and then go on to imply that it will be possible to develop interventions to suit all these various experiences, that can then be evaluated in terms that will be relevant across the world.

Again, the links between academic theorizing and professional practice are potentially highly significant, with the theoretical underpinnings of 'adolescence' being very apparent in the professional literature and practice, such that this theoretical framework could be said to have become institutionalized.[2] Indeed, Wyn and White (1997: 34) argue that developmental theories serve to legitimize institutional processes which 'systematically marginalise, fail or exclude particular groups of young people'. Other researchers (e.g. Alderson and Montgomery 1996) have provided us with insights into the ways in which 'developmental' phases that appear to be based

---

[2] There are parallels here with the ways in which the professional training of teachers is still very heavily based in psychological theories of child development, despite the publication in recent years of considerable bodies of academic work that offer an alternative approach to theorizing childhood (see Chapter 1). See Rose (1989) for further discussion of the ways in which the 'psy' discourses have become heavily institutionalized in western societies over the last two centuries, and Small and Hockey (2001) for a discussion of a Foucauldian perspective in relation to grief and bereavement.

in chronological age may actually be heavily modified by specific relevant experiences.

While these psychological approaches may be found to have value in the context of professional practice in contemporary western societies, there is clearly scope for much further exploration and theorizing about the potential significance of bereavement in relation to the teenage years, building on the more sociological approaches that view youth as an age status that is socially constructed. Such an alternative approach might yield further insights and understandings of the lives of young people that may also be valuable for professional practices, particularly across different social contexts, taking into account the extent to which youth is cross-cut by other key sources of socially structured differences. Nevertheless, we would not want to overstate the divergence between these theoretical and disciplinary approaches, nor present them as inevitably dualistic. It is clear that some of the existing work in this area does indeed draw on both theoretical frameworks, even if only implicitly.

One predominant feature of sociological and social policy approaches to the lives of young people has been a reliance on the concept of 'transition' (Gillies 2001). The supposed transition between childhood and adulthood is, however, argued to have become increasingly multifarious and complex in contemporary western societies, with some transitions having become elongated while others have become truncated (Jones 2002, 2005), leading to a situation of disarray and confusion. A rather different approach is suggested by Wyn and White (1997: 11), who argue that:

> Youth ... is most usefully seen as a *relational* concept, which refers to the social processes whereby age is socially constructed, institutionalised and controlled in historically and culturally specific ways ... Youth is a relational concept because it exists and has meaning largely in relation to the concept of adulthood ... youth is a state of 'becoming' [and] adulthood is the 'arrival'.

These writers do go on, however, to consider whether cultural ideas about 'youth' are becoming increasingly detached from age status *per se* (discussed further below).

Exploiting the potential of such alternative approaches to theorizing the teenage years is beyond our remit here, but we can perhaps point to some possibilities concerning the ways in which key themes in youth studies could be linked to bereavement issues. Some of the core debates in this literature on youth (see e.g. Furlong and Cartmel 1997; Wyn and White 1997; Brannen *et al.* 2002), have centred around a variety of topics (some of which clearly overlap or interrelate):

- various institutionalized transitional experiences, particularly educational, economic and labour market transitions;
- youth cultures, including a variety of aspects such as risk-taking, deviance, sexuality, media, drug use, neighbourhood and locality;
- leisure, lifestyle and consumption;
- health behaviours, both physical and mental;
- identities and development;
- the development of intimacy, including pregnancy and parenthood;
- peer groups;
- 'family' relationships.

In the context of bereavement, there are clear possibilities for links between such issues, in terms, for example, of the themes of risk, identity, the body, deviance, peer groups and significant relationships, which potentially point to a variety of types of bereavement such as suicide, drug-related deaths, miscarriage and abortion, accidental deaths, violent deaths, as well as the development of links with the more recognized issues of parental or sibling bereavement.

In the social policy arena (which interrelates closely with sociological literature, but may also draw on the more psychological approaches – e.g. see Bynner *et al.* 1997; Barry 2004), young people's position may be framed in variable ways, with differing implications for bereavement issues:

- as students in relation to educational issues;
- as future citizens in the context of citizenship education;
- as current citizens in terms of rights and social exclusion;
- as consumers in relation to the self-help and therapeutic literatures.

One key theme that has been identified in relation to the family lives of young people is a significant ambiguity about young people as moral agents. Children have been argued to be outside of moral accountability in contemporary western societies (Ribbens McCarthy and Edwards 2000), while adulthood is understood as requiring moral accountability. One aspect of the status of youth, then, is a complex and uncertain position in terms of whether or not a young person is seen as morally accountable in her or his own right, both in relation to the care of others and the care of self. Thus, while adults may perceive the teenage years in terms of a growing independence, understood as a freedom to make their own choices, young people themselves may see such independence as entailing a growing responsibility (Gillies *et al.* 2001).

The freedom to be self-determining thus carries the cost of having to take (moral) responsibility for one's self, which includes the sort of stringent requirements for self-control of the body and emotions that Elias (2000) and Featherstone (1995) discuss (as outlined below), which in turn poses particular issues to do with risk-taking for young people as they acquire such new experiences of freedom and responsibility. Teenagers in western societies have to move from childhood non-responsibility to a position of responsibility via self-control. This may provide an insight, therefore, into issues of drugs and drink (for example) as a way of resisting this sort of imperative for self-control and responsibility for one's own (changing) body, by contrast with issues like anorexia which involve an excessive state of control of one's own body. It is arguable, then, that the body itself has a particular significance during the teenage years because of the ways in which we have constructed childhood, adulthood and the transition between them. Young people may be exploring the limits, possibilities, advantages and disadvantages of (loss of) control of the body, and this may implicate particular meanings to do with death, which so crucially centralizes understandings of what the body signifies. Similarly, one could develop particular arguments about how emotions, and connections with others via both bodies and emotions, are likely to be particular foci of concern during the transitions of youth (discussed further in Chapter 5). In these various ways, young people may be 'testing out' the limits of reality and the possible consequences (Holland 2002), and death and bereavement may indeed have a particular significance in this context.

While the responsibility for managing the potential disruptiveness of children is seen to lie with parents or adult care-takers (Ribbens McCarthy and Edwards 2002), this responsibility is diffused in the teenage years, leading to fears about teenagers as potentially disruptive without anyone being clearly responsible or in control. Teenagers may thus be stereotyped in various ways as: potentially threatening (through disruption and loss of control); a source of optimism (hope for the future); or victims (through their marginal social status).

An emphasis on the teenage years as an institutionally-based age status opens up the question of what young people may be seen to have in common. This may be understood (Wyn and White 1997) in terms of:

- a shared administrative and bureaucratic category;
- a clearly identified target for consumer markets and media;
- a problematic labour market situation;
- an ambiguous financial standing.

Such a view then poses questions about the social position of youth as carrying certain implications for the negotiation or assertion of power. This may be particularly relevant to a consideration of bereavement in the lives of young people, since a key feature of bereavement can be a significantly heightened sense of vulnerability. Bereavement and grief thus relate to general issues about how we deal with vulnerability in public and private, and in the context of differing power relations. This then points to issues about how death, dying and bereavement are understood and socially mediated in contemporary western societies.

Theorizing death and dying

Death and dying have become the focus of a very substantial body of academic (particularly historical and sociological) work, which theorizes how death is understood in the conditions of high- or post-modernity.[3] Such understandings of death, formulated in the specific sociohistorical contexts of contemporary western societies, underpin the literatures on bereavement that have been developed in these contexts, as well as how individual young people may experience bereavement in their lives.

The work of the social historian Ariés (1974, 1981) in this area has been path-breaking, if sometimes controversial and disputed (e.g. see Elias 1985). Through the analysis of historical documents and architecture, Ariés saw changes in the attitude to death in western societies, between the middle ages and the nineteenth century. These include:

- the development of 'a sense of personal and specific biography' (Ariés 1981: 609);
- exclusion of death within society due to death becoming a secular and medical event that was viewed as 'dirty', requiring removal to sanitized and hygienic hospitals;
- increasing privatization of death within the family, associated with a rejection of ritualized, public ceremony.

For Ariés, from this time on, death was denied and effectively driven into secrecy, until the second half of the twentieth century.

The late nineteenth and early twentieth centuries also saw a particularly marked and widespread change in mortality rates (Anderson 1990), leading to

---

[3] These terms of high- or post-modernity are ones that are keenly debated in sociological theory, but the details of these debates are not crucial here. The differences may be roughly summarized by reference to (a) Giddens's (1990) assertion of the nature of modernity in terms of a post-Enlightenment project of continual development and progress through the onward march of rational secularized thought and knowledge, having led into (b) a period of high modernity (in Giddens's view) in which we see new developments that are nevertheless fundamentally based on the accentuation and extension of these earlier principles, as against (c) the alternative argument (e.g. as posited by Bauman 1997) that we have moved into a period of post-modernity, in which the rational project of modernity has been challenged and seen to have broken down, leading to complexity, contradiction, and a loss of the meta-narrative of progress.

a change in the predominant age of death, from the young to the old, and a new association of death with ageing, such that youth and death may be seen as categories that are not expected to coincide. Other associated changes have included an increase in the public bureaucratization of death (Armstrong 1987), through the development of death registration processes. Other writers, including sociologists and anthropologists (see Hockey 1990; Field 1996), have argued that the distancing of death from everyday experiences (as first described by Ariés), has led to a view of death and dying as the province of specialists, whose expertise is rationalized, medicalized and secularized. Death has thus been described as a public absence/private presence (Mellor 1993). Indeed, some writers suggest that, in a cross-cultural perspective, contemporary western cultures have more time limited, and less elaborate, death rituals than many other societies (Rosenblatt 2001, discussed further below). Furthermore, it is argued that 'Western cultures, which tend to discourage the overt expression of emotion at funerals, are highly deviant. They differ from most other societies and from our own society as it was a hundred years ago' (Parkes *et al.* 1997: 5). Some writers suggest that this may in part at least be associated with the experiences of the two world wars (Walter 1999).

Giddens (1990, 1991) extends such arguments to wider processes of the 'sequestration' of experience in high modernity. While death is said to have been 'bracketed out' of contemporary western societies, as lying outside modern principles of order, control and rationality, conditions of high modernity have led to radical doubt and questioning about knowledge and the foundations of meta-narratives (which could be taken to include religious understandings of the meaning of death and suffering). Meaning has become privatized, as everyone is compelled to make sense of their everyday lives themselves, such that young people, too, may view themselves as responsible for shaping their own destinies (Furlong and Cartmel 1997). This meaning is fragile and open to continual threat, leading to a fundamental problem of the potential for personal meaninglessness, associated with a continual search for the achievement of 'ontological security'. At the same time, the most challenging moral questions remain avoided and unanswered, with the quintissential removal of death from everyday experience via the medicalized and institutionalized framework of the hospital.

Such historical developments are seen to have culminated in new debates about how to manage death in the mid-twentieth century. Elias (1985) has argued that the main difficulty for the dying is the loneliness they experience as they die away from their communities in institutional environments and, when visited, with no formal rituals to rely on, people no longer know what to say or do. The intervention of medicine was argued to have had a dehumanizing effect on the experience of death and dying, and such debates led to new, psychosocial, professional discourses about the stages of dying and of bereavement (Kubler-Ross 1969, 1981). These debates about the costs and benefits of medical processes were associated in the 1960s with institutional changes in the form of the hospice movement and associated bereavement counselling services (Small and Hockey 2001), as well as the development of new specialisms within medicine, such as palliative care nursing, that sought to rethink and modify some of the existing medical practices. These debates continue and are associated with ongoing, and ambivalent, tensions between medical and therapeutic discourses and practices.

More recent sociological theorizing concerned with the social processes of post-modernity has led to suggestions that death is being deconstructed via an emphasis on bodies and survival strategies, such that death (in small ways) is seen to be pervasive but controllable through survival strategies of self-care and lifestyle (Bauman 1992a, 1992b, 1998). Seale (1998: 193) argues that everyday life and micro-interactions constitute mundane experiences of loss and its repair, in turn constituting 'small psychic losses, exclusions and humiliations, alternating with moments of repair and optimism' (1998: 193). In these ways, we may become preoccupied with the continual task of postponing death through vigilance about health, a task which entails a daily rehearsal of mortality through its everyday practice (Bauman 1992a, 1992b). The paradox, however, is that this is a battle that, in the ultimate sense, can only be postponed and never won.

The ways in which consumer cultures intersect with these processes have been examined by Featherstone (1995), who argues that we have come to celebrate the virtues of youth, self-preservation and the beautiful body. Consumer culture, however, has only contradictory solutions to the problem of death. Death and dying have to be hidden away to ensure we can maintain the illusion of the good life here and now. At the same time, the fear of death and dying has to be promoted to ensure individuals are vigilant in their self-care and body maintenance regimes, around which consumer markets may be built. Such issues may be writ particularly large in the lives of young people, since ' "Youth" now has symbolic value as the "outcome" of the process of becoming more and more in control over one's body' (Wyn and White 1997: 20). Furthermore, Wyn and White argue, the meaning of 'youth' has the potential to become detached from age, to signify the possibility of 'being anything you want to be' (p. 21) – a theme which, Craib (1994) suggests, may have become central to contemporary western cultures.

At the same time, widespread (news and fictional) media coverage of death, bereavement and grief provides a sense of being intimately acquainted with such experiences (Walter 1991), but such media glimpses of distant experiences, in which bodily experiences continue to be hidden from view, may prove irrelevant to direct personal experiences of the death of loved ones. There are thus many contradictions and tensions when considering the role of the media, particularly in the context of young people. For example, in the USA it is estimated that children have witnessed several thousand fictional deaths before the teenage years (Katz 2001). This then raises further major issues about how young people relate to, and use, media in the context of their own lives.

The core value of rationality that is theorized to underlie the sequestration of death is also seen to underpin the ways in which western cultures have become increasingly individualized. The 'civilizing processes' (Elias 2000) of modernity are linked to a view of the rational (Adult) individual, who can bring disorderly emotions and behaviour under conscious control, avoiding chaotic and unmannerly disruptions to public social contexts (concerns which we can see writ large in the context of youth in public places). Emotions become the particular province of an individualized 'inner world', risking a sense of emotional isolation, an isolation which is intensified in relation to the emotions of grief by the decline in public mourning rituals (Ariés 1974, 1981). Walter (1999) suggests that such processes of individualization in relation to experiences of death, dying and mourning may be increasing, as evidenced by emergent practices concerned with the individualization of funerals. Seale (1998) however, drawing on the work of Bourdieu, argues that these experiences may constitute important features of a social capital that is not equally available to all sectors of the community, with issues of class, ethnicity and gender creating further dimensions to these processes.

Death and dying may also be individualized in relation to the death of the body, at least as this is understood within the context of the contemporary western medical and bureaucratic frameworks discussed above. It can also (but need not necessarily – see Miller 1997) be taken to refer to the ultimate personal journey of the individual, taken alone, which irrevocably severs all mortal connections, the ultimate individualized biographical narrative. Walter (1999) argues that there has been a development of the ideal type of post-modern death, in which the authority of the individual is paramount, to make choices and control the dying process. As public expert discourses are challenged and fragmented, the private is celebrated. This raises further questions, however, as to the extent to which people do, in practice, have such choices, and how this issue may be cross-cut by gender, age status, class and ethnicity (Field *et al.* 1997).

Seale (1998: 201) argues that western societies have developed processes of social death that anticipate physical death through 'compulsory disengagement', for example, through retirement or institutional care, such that 'in late modern society there is a general aspiration towards anticipatory grief, so that mourning in large part then occurs before a person dies ... leaving little to grieve for after this event'. The notion of 'anticipatory grief' has also become the focus of developments in theorizing and practices of grief in the medicalized literature (Small and Hockey 2001). Seale's work, however, like Hockey's (1990), is largely concerned with deaths of aged people. Whether or not his assertion holds true in such contexts, it seems doubtful that there is empirical evidence to support this generalization where the deaths of younger people are concerned. In the context of youth, death may be seen as a shocking and inappropriate intrusion, as death 'out of time'.

Concepts of bereavement, grief and mourning

Unlike (individualized) concepts of death and dying, bereavement always implicates a *relationship* of some sort, since there can be no bereavement outside the context of a relationship. Bereavement through death can refer to a great range of such relationships, from death of a parent or sibling to the demise of a pet, from the death of a grandparent to an abortion. Among the various sociological writers, Walter (1991, 1999) has paid the most extended attention to bereavement in this sense (while Small and Hockey 2001 offer a combination of sociological and anthropological insights). Walter argues that bereaved people constitute anomalies in western rational societies, subjected to social processes of both regulation and integration, and located at the boundaries of life and death. Bereaved people are thus faced with (individualized) dilemmas, firstly of how to relate to the dead (are they meant to 'let go' or not?), and secondly of how to relate to the living (are they meant to control their emotions or express their grief, and in what contexts?). Such anomalies may be associated with increasing specialization of discourses and organized services for bereaved people (Small and Hockey 2001), which deal with bereavement as a particular and troubling experience, outside the general context of the beginning and ending of relationships more broadly.

Seale is another sociologist who also makes important theoretical points about bereavement, although his primary focus is on death and dying. His primary thesis concerns the centrality of the social bond for human living, such that grief can be understood as 'a reaction to extreme damage to the social bond' (1998: 193). He argues that loss threatens our personal ontological security because it undermines our social bond, and he uses the concept of 'resurrection' to refer to the 'hope in survivors about continuing in life' (p. 194). This may have particular resonance for the lives of young people who may be in process of renegotiating existing social relationships and also building new ones.

Seale also argues that grief, like death, has been heavily medicalized in western discourses and practices, leading to 'its depiction as a disease' (1998: 195). This may be understood as a feature of 'the medical profession's tendency to view all human distress as explainable in medical terms and treatable by medical means, and the willingness of the laity to believe that this is so' (Seale 2001: 46). Small and Hockey take this sort of argument further, using a Foucauldian analysis to suggest that discourses of bereavement and grief can serve to extend the social regulation or 'policing' (Walter 1999) of internal emotions. Indeed, Small and Hockey (2001: 107) suggest that 'the grieving process can be differentiated from mourning in that it is increasingly the bereaved person's internal world, rather than an external social environment, which constitutes the site for activity and change'.

The sociologist and psychoanalyst Ian Craib (1994) suggests that the development of such expert forms of knowledge and guidance reflects the wider trend for modern societies to seek to avoid confronting the inevitability of human pain, suffering and 'the full terror of disappointment' (p. 28). Expert interventions, he argues, thus aim to control mourning and cover it up as much as possible. The result is 'shallow' accounts and interpretations of grief as feelings, rather than as the deep-rooted internal processing of experience at an unconscious level. At the same time, he suggests, some of the difficulties of grief have been created by modern society in the first place, by having no socially recognized period of 'functional impairment'. Furthermore, if we cannot tolerate pain and suffering, and rely instead on a belief in the resolution of grief through expert guidance, we may draw out a false self that cannot deal with the destructive processes of late modernity.

Outside these sociological academic debates – and very disconnected from them – there is an extensive literature on bereavement as a particular form of loss, along with the associated terms of grief and mourning. These terms have multiple meanings (Katz 2001) and may sometimes be used in quite inconsistent and even contradictory ways, but the nature of these definitions generally does support Small and Hockey's assertion (above) that grief is defined as 'internal', while mourning is defined as 'external'. Drawing on Raphael (1984 discussed by Small 2001b), we may initially define these terms as follows:

- bereavement as 'the process of losing a close relationship' through death;
- mourning as 'the period of time during which signs of grief are made visible', often referring to social and cultural practices concerned with grief rather than the individual processes implied by grief and bereavement;
- grief as 'the pain and suffering experienced after loss'; and
- loss as 'the state of being deprived of, or being without, something one has had' (Small 2001b: 20).

All of these terms are 'culturally mediated' and 'socially understood' (Katz 2001: 4; see also Seale 1998; Walter 1999). These definitions, however, raise questions (explored in more detail below) about how far bereavement is always, and unequivocally, a loss, and whether loss is always, and unequivocally, associated with negative experiences and outcomes.

Grief can thus be described as the response or reaction to loss, and may be viewed as 'an activity rather than a state of being' (Katz 2001: 5). It is often taken to refer to the emotional content of bereavement, although it is also clear (as can be seen in the opening quote from Virginia Ironside on p. ix) that lay understandings of grief are often quite narrowly framed around pain, rather than the broader array of possible emotions that Ironside describes. Grief may also be linked to the term 'work', understood in the therapeutic sense of 'working' on oneself, as in references to 'grief work' as 'a process of learning' and a 'psychosocial transition' (Parkes 1998, discussed in Katz 2001). Framing grief as 'work' can lead on to notions of 'techniques' that can be used as tools in this process (Small and Hockey 2001).

All of these terms are relevant to our focus of interest here, but in different ways and with variable implications:

- Is it useful to see bereavement within an overarching framework of 'loss' or 'change', in which case we will perceive continuities with other forms of experience in the lives of young people, or is there something particular about bereavement – or at least some bereavements – that mark it as presenting a particular and different experience at the level of individual experiences and biographies of young people?
- What nature of bereavement might we be considering here? Are we only concerned with loss through death of 'close' or significant relationships, and if so, how can we identify these in research terms? What sorts of relationship might young people be at risk of losing through death? We could, for example, be primarily talking about 'family' relationships, such as parents, siblings and grandparents. But we could also be talking about the death of lovers, partners, unborn children, friends, acquaintances and even pets. Can such a wide potential array of bereavements be objectively and empirically operationalized in ways that allow us to produce relevant research findings, or is bereavement too subjective an experience to allow for this?
- How far is it helpful to understand grief as a matter of highly individualized emotional responses to bereavement, a matter of the interior life of the young person – albeit often theorized as showing certain universal processual commonalities – or do we need scope to understand grief as embedded in specific social contexts which may present different expectations and frameworks of meaning for such emotional responses? How far does the socially defined age category of 'youth' present one such relevant social context? Do we also, however, need to consider the experiences of bereaved young people as systematically patterned by reference to gender, class, ethnicity, or other aspects of social structures and cultures?

- Is mourning, as a set of ritualized and visible social practices, irrelevant to the experiences of bereaved young people in contemporary Britain? Does mourning refer to practices that are situated in the more 'public' social settings, and if so, are young people faced with declining social practices for making their grief visible, such that they are left dealing with it at a very 'private' level? Do we have any socially structured frameworks by which young people may deal with grief at a social level? How do these questions relate to the experiences of young people in their educational, family and peer group contexts?

Theorizing bereavement and grief

Associated with the denial of death theories discussed earlier, in the 1960s Gorer (1987) suggested that people in the UK no longer knew how to grieve. However, since the mid-twentieth century there has been a significant growth in the literature about loss and bereavement. This literature may, in the light of sociological theories of death, dying and bereavement in high or post-modernity (discussed above), perhaps be understood as attempts to provide some secular order and control out of the experienced chaos of death and grief. Seale (1998: 11) asserts that nature, in the form of the death of the body, which symbolizes the ultimate limits of culture, represents 'meaningless chaos' (resonating with views of loss as a crisis of meaning, discussed in Chapter 1). Building on the work of the anthropologist Mary Douglas, Seale suggests that classificatory thinking (of which theories of the stages of grief may be taken as an example) constitutes 'the imposition of order upon disorder, which is a bracketing out of existential dread through the cultural construction of everyday regimes' (p. 160). Nevertheless, other anthropologists (notably Strathern 1992) might suggest that 'nature' itself is constructed in particular ways by contemporary western cultures, such that understandings of death itself may be seen as naturalised, even while 'nature' itself is socially constructed.

Parkes (discussed in Walter 1999) has distinguished between three models to summarize the scientific approach to grief (all of which have been scrutinized and criticized, and which are not necessarily mutually exclusive):

1 The processes of grief that are classified within the *phase model.*
2 The effort that is required to make sense of, and make the loss real, within the grief *work model.*
3 The association of grief as an illness/'disease' within the *medical model.*

The theories or assumptions that underpin these various grief models are in turn based on various theories of psychoanalysis or psychosocial processes, such as Freud's work on cathexis and mourning, Klein's work on object relations theory, Bowlby's work on attachment and loss and Parkes' work on psychosocial transitions.

The first model listed above refers to a theoretical understanding of grief that built on the work of Kubler-Ross (1969, 1981) in relation to the process of dying. This model suggests that grief entails a fairly linear progression through various *phases or stages* – shock and denial, pining, reorganization and recovery (entailing a 'letting go' of the lost loved one) (see e.g. Raphael 1984; Gorer 1987). This theoretical perspective has become an established basis for professional training and self-help literature in the field of bereavement.

Whatever model is taken of 'the grief process', there may also be the assertion of an associated requirement for *grief 'work'* to be undertaken, if the bereavement is to lead to some sort of resolution. In relation to parentally bereaved children, this view sees grief as a set of tasks in terms of 'normal responses' (Worden 1996: 16). Worden discusses the tasks as being: to accept the reality of death; to deal with the emotional impact of the loss; to adjust to an environment in which the deceased is absent; and to emotionally relocate the deceased. He suggests that these tasks can be dealt with in any order, and may vary according to the age and developmental level of the child. In the context of the lives of young people, this approach has been further elaborated by reference to what are theorized as the developmental tasks of adolescence (discussed further below), the aim being to achieve a 'healthy' rather than a 'pathological' outcome, i.e. a *medical model*.

Various criticisms may be levelled at these models, criticisms which may at times point to intrinsic features of these theories, while in other cases they may suggest limitations in the ways in which the theories have been presented, which could be resolved by further modifications or re-framing. Most fundamentally, such models may be accused of asserting an unfounded universalism as to the nature of grief and its associated emotionality, and of failing to consider differences, whether these concern broad cultural differences, or variations associated with structural differences such as age status, gender, class or ethnicity. Linked to this charge of universalism is the assertion that these models are closely associated with the medicalization of grief (see Seale 1998). This may be constructed in psychiatric terms, in that the person may require active intervention to progress through to adjustment and acceptance (possibly in terms of a 'successful bereavement').

The association of grief with physical processes (fatigue, breathlessness, tenseness etc.) and the association of grief with ill health may also be linked with the medicalized view of bereavement, which points to the way in which grief became constructed as a 'disease' – with the differentiation between normal and pathological. From this perspective, much research may be concerned to specify the indicators for 'pathological', or, more recently, for 'complicated' grief (Prigerson 2005), as distinct from 'normal' grief reactions.[4] In relation to young people specifically, however, Ayers *et al.* (2003), drawing on the work of Stroebe *et al.*, suggest that we have very little work available to make such distinctions with any confidence. Finally, within the psychiatric discourse, grief is 'hard work', a struggle of the inner self, but there is a reward for the bereaved as they eventually return to a form of normality.

The medicalized/therapeutic approach thus privileges the individual body and the 'inner world' in relation to the sociocultural context of bereavement, so that, for example, our understanding of bereavement may now relate to the extent that we are seen to be successful at passing through the stages of grief. One therapeutic approach that does explicitly look beyond the individual is that based on family systemic theorizing (see e.g. Bowlby-West 1983; Sutcliffe *et al.* 1998; McBride and Simms 2001), but such theories have themselves also been accused of operating on a restricted set of assumptions about how family relationships may be defined and understood as 'healthy' or 'dysfunctional' in ways that may mask ethnocentric, or other culturally mediated, assumptions (see e.g. Dilworth-Anderson *et al.* 1993). Small and Hockey (2001: 112) suggest that, while such family systemic models of grief widen out the narrow focus from the individual, the implications for practice remain the same, since 'It is the family, rather than the individual, who is still presented with "tasks"'.

More recently, however, some alternative (though still generally very individualized) models have been presented and have received a good deal of support, even if they have not been centralized in professional training. The first of these newer, more complex models is that of the *dual process approach* to loss (Stroebe and Schut 1995, 1999), discussed by Riches and Dawson (2000) and Thompson (2002). This model theorizes grief over time as associated with a continuing oscillation between the loss orientation of grief and the restoration orientation to continuity of living. Such an approach is in line with recent discussion of the goal of 'coping' with bereavement rather than finding a 'resolution' of grief (Corr 2000a). Thompson (2002: 7) argues that this dual process model 'alerts us to the complex web of psychological, cultural and sociopolitical factors which interact to make loss experiences far more complex than traditional approaches would have us believe'.

There are two further shifts in perspective that Thompson outlines, and which he suggests can be usefully combined with the dual process model.

---

[4] For a sociological critique of such measurement scales, see Small (2001a). Craib argues that concepts of pathological grief may be in the eye of the beholder, and queries whether varying reactions to bereavement should be taken as indicators of pathology, or of a 'different soul' (1994: 29).

One concerns the move away from the orthodoxy that grief has to involve a process of 'letting go' before it can be resolved, to one which sees the presence of *continuing bonds* as being compatible with a restoration orientation (Klass *et al.* 1996; Walter 1999).

The second emergent perspective that Thompson discusses is that of *meaning reconstruction theory* (Neimeyer 2001; Neimeyer and Anderson 2002). This theory views the loss of meaning as fundamental to the experience of loss, such that 'meaning reconstruction in response to loss is the central feature of grieving', a process which is 'deeply personal and intricately social' (Neimeyer and Anderson 2002: 47). Such reconstruction of meaning may encompass practical, existential and spiritual narrative themes, which are, at least partially, based on shared cultural meanings. Narrative is central to the reconstruction of meaning but Neimeyer and Anderson suggest that this is not seen as purely a cognitive process, but 'an impassioned effort to find sustaining meanings that offer new and practical reorientation in our world with others' (p. 49). Drawing on the work of Attig, Neimeyer and Anderson argue (p. 50) that grief requires us to 'relearn the self' and 'relearn the world'. (We consider narrative approaches further in Chapter 3, in the context of our case studies, and we return to issues of 'meaning' in Chapter 6.)

As Thompson points out, this approach also resonates with the 'progressive-regressive' method of existentialist theory. There are also, we might add, further resonances with more sociological work, including that which takes an interpretivist or constructivist approach, such as that of Seale (1998, discussed above), and also the work of Marris (1996), in which he suggests that 'meaning' is the central way in which we attempt to deal with the inevitable uncertainty that is 'a fundamental condition of human life' (p. 1). Marris also seeks to link the individual search for meaning with an analysis of the cultural availability of meanings and the processes of power that shape the ability to control uncertainty.

A rather different categorization of theories of grief is offered by Riches and Dawson (2000). They classify models as representing conventional approaches, new understandings, or systems approaches. Within the new understandings they include humanistic approaches, which see bereavement as a particular example of life crisis which can provide opportunities for personal learning given empathetic support. They also offer their own approach, drawing on identity theory to define bereavement as 'the damage to identity caused by the loss of a relationship that is central to a personal sense of self and purpose' (p. 12). Such an emphasis on identity can draw on both sociological and psychological theoretical frameworks, including those that view identity formation as a key issue for adolescent development (discussed further below).

As indicated in Chapter 1, where we raised issues about the reflexivity of the knowledge production process, and the ways in which expert theories may interconnect with 'popular' understandings of bereavement and grief, the theories of grief outlined above may resonate in diverse ways with (highly variable) lay understandings of everyday experiences of bereavement in daily life, and managing grief in various social contexts. Through written texts, media presentations and professional interactions, 'expert' theories and 'clinical lore' (Walter 1999) may become available as 'discourses' that people draw upon when seeking to find some sense of order or meaning in their individual bereavement experiences. People may then also draw upon such discourses when interviewed for research purposes, constituting a mutually reinforcing circle of knowledge production and affirmation.

Nevertheless, these discourses may be disseminated to varying degrees among different social groups, and may be countered by discourses of longer standing, based in the cultures of everyday lives. Small and Hockey (2001) also discuss the ways in which mutual self-help groups may create a type of 'counter culture' to such expert discourses. Walter (1999) suggests that two main positions may be discerned with regard to such 'lay' interpretations and understandings of bereavement and grief in the contemporary UK context: one is that the emotions of grief should be contained, especially in public, and distraction is a useful way of overcoming grief, while the second, more therapeutically inclined, view is that grief should be expressed and talked through to aid recovery. This latter view has been questioned (Walter 1999; Riches 2002) as privileging women's experience of grief in terms of the emphasis on the emotional expression of grief (and we return to debates about the value of talk in Chapter 5).

However, this leads us on to further issues about the sorts of research evidence available concerning such 'lay' or 'everyday' discourses of grief and bereavement. While the theories of bereavement and grief (such as those of Raphael 1984) that have been outlined here may have been based on the careful and extended observations of, and clinical involvement with, individual bereaved people, there are questions that may be raised about how far this constitutes a satisfactory basis for the development of models that have been so widely used and applied. There may thus be further scope for other ways of researching and analysing everyday experiences of bereavement and grief. These issues will be explored in more detail in Chapter 3, in relation to young people's experiences of, and perspectives on, death and bereavement.

'Bereavement', 'loss' and 'change'

'Loss' as a term may be seen to be rooted in the theorizing of either Freud (through his work on cathexis) or Bowlby (through his work on attachment and separation). In a Freudian perspective, loss and its associated griefs are

never retrievable, while Bowlby's consideration of loss is rooted in his theories of attachment, and may have more scope for viewing the associated
grief as resolvable at some level. As a concept it is clearly much broader than
that of bereavement, and may refer to a great variety of different sorts of
experiences, over quite variable time periods (Katz 2001). It is a term that is
frequently linked with bereavement (and may in some literatures – as well as
in everyday conversations – be used in place of bereavement), often with the
explicit aim of pointing to the continuities between bereavement experiences and other experiences of loss, continuities which may be seen as
helpful for practitioners (Murray, 2001). These might encompass, for example, family changes such as divorce, other sorts of lifestyle changes, such
as moving house or school, or more psychic changes, such as loss of identity,
self-esteem or role – these latter particularly being seen as potentially relevant during the teenage years (Doka 2000). However, while such connections between loss and bereavement may be made in the literatures, they are
not always carried through in any detail, which probably reflects the en-
ormity of the potential issues that are thus opened up. The collection edited
by Doka (2000), for example, which is subtitled *Children, Adolescents and
Loss*, after the initial discussion, actually includes chapters that are all about
loss through death.[5]

How helpful is the term 'loss', then, to our understanding of bereavement
experiences? As outlined above, the concept of 'bereavement' is largely to be
found in a particular literature that is rooted in counselling and other therapeutic interventions. 'Loss', on the other hand, is a term that is widely used
in the social work literature. While Craib (1994) argues from a psychoanalytic
perspective that loss is central to infant development, as a concept, 'loss'
points to the deprivation of something that *had* been present, that has been
taken away or is *no longer there*. 'Loss' thus risks being understood as constituting a deficit with inherent negative connotations, unlike, perhaps, the
more neutral concept of 'change'. If the object of your attachment disappears
(or at least, becomes transformed, e.g. the woman I married to the woman I
divorced) then it almost becomes tautological that this disappearance will
constitute a loss. Corr (2000a: 28), for example, points to 'loss' as entailing
'harm' by its linkage with something that is 'valued': 'When anyone experiences the loss of someone or some thing that is valued, he or she is harmed'.

Whether or not bereavement constitutes a 'loss' in this sense is likely to
be highly variable, dependent on the level and nature of the attachment
rather than the category of the deceased. If the relationship was not

---

[5] But see Thompson (2002) for an edited collection which does cover a variety of
substantive issues within the theoretical framework of 'loss', including divorce, adop-
tion and foster care, disability, ill health, ageing, and justice.

particularly significant, or even experienced quite negatively, bereavement will not have the same meaning as where the relationship was very central and positive to the bereaved person's life. At the same time, however, the death of someone who is a significant if difficult part of one's life may still be associated with strong emotions, even if the grief experience may be less central (as indicated by the opening quote by Ironside on p. ix). Alternatively, if the attachment was largely circumstantial and fortuitous, its loss might provide different opportunities for new attachments, as in the example of the young man who fails his exams but then embarks on a different career that he later regards as having opened up different but beneficial opportunities. Again, if the attachment is understood (perhaps by others) to have been positively detrimental to our well-being (in some respects at least), then the consequent feelings of loss may be seen to some degree as 'inappropriate' (resulting in a 'disenfranchised grief', Doka 2000 discussed by Thompson 2002), as in the case of the young girl who loses (what others consider to be) a very undesirable boyfriend, or who terminates a very early pregnancy.

Besides such issues as the nature of the attachment or prior relationship, the experience of bereavement may also depend on a variety of contextual issues and factors, including, for example, other material, social and psychological resources available; the extent to which it constitutes one of multiple sources of difficulty in a person's life; the extent to which they have prior experiences that may help them make sense of it; and the degree to which it is experienced as leading to a sense of disruption and isolation (discussed further in subsequent chapters). Some of these factors might be expected to work in opposite ways in different contexts. For example, we know that mortality rates and ages of death have been, and continue to be, significantly related to social class and material inequalities that are geographically located in contemporary Britain (see Chapter 1), so that the death of a parent might be more commonly experienced, and therefore shared, in more working-class neighbourhoods, potentially providing readier sources of support and understanding than might be the case in a more affluent community. For a middle-class teenager, therefore, the death of a parent may be experienced as a more unusual and unknown individual trauma, but on the other hand, the likelihood of greater financial resources (in the form of life insurance and other forms of capital) may serve to reduce the degree of consequent disruption. Evidence does suggest that such issues of local context can be notably related to issues both of familiarity with death and bereavement, and also fears of dying oneself (Morin and Welsh 1996; Holland 2002), although for different reasons in different localities.

This discussion, then, raises issues about how far the theoretical underpinnings of such key concepts as loss and bereavement provide scope for seeing a death as anything other than painful, undesirable and destructive. As a society, perhaps we grow ever more fearful of pain – whether physical or emotional – only ever seeing it as something to be avoided (Craib 1994). Is there scope for seeing some pain as productive and creative (Frantz *et al.* 2001)? We raise this question, not in the rather crass sense of suggesting that 'bereavement' may be seen as a learning opportunity, or an opportunity for 'growth' (although some bereaved people might themselves argue for this)[6] but, rather, to seek to maintain a conceptual and theoretical space that will allow any particular bereavement to be seen as complex and ambiguous. In this respect, then, we hope not to jump to any premature conclusions of bereavement as always constituting a (negative) loss, or always problematic in any simplistic way. But, while Craib (1994) argues for a complex and imperfect (psychoanalytic) account of pain and grief, other authors do write quite unequivocally of the potential for bereavement and loss to lead to positive benefits. Corr and McNeil (1986: 77), for example, write that 'By learning to cope in an effective manner with loss and death, adolescents enhance the quality of their own lives and the lives of those with whom they come into contact'. Balk (1995: 175), in similar vein, writes that 'a paradoxical aspect of life crises is that they can promote growth and maturity while at the same time threatening dysfunction and dissolution'.

The extent to which bereavement has to be understood as a subjective experience, which can only very roughly be captured by any sort of objective empirical operationalization in terms, for example, of the category of relationship involved in the bereavement, is perhaps partly why sociologists have tended to avoid using the concept. However, some of the newer fields of sociology, particularly the sociology of emotions, may open up new ways of approaching such issues, providing further insights into the ways in which emotions surrounding bereavement, whether of grief or not, may be socially mediated and contextualized, or even 'produced' (Small and Hockey 2001). We return later to the possibilities of new synergies between different disciplinary perspectives in this area, but next we turn to consider more directly how we might understand the conjunction of 'young people' and 'bereavement' in relation to the possible time trajectories involved.

Young people and the trajectory of time

As mentioned earlier, we set out on this project using an open-ended approach to how we might operationalize the term 'young people', to refer to the teenage years and early twenties. What this inevitably connotes, however, is a time trajectory (although, as Small 2001a discusses, the experience of

---

[6] Eisenstadt (1978) has argued that parental loss is linked to genius in adulthood, as well as with psychosis.

bereavement may itself fracture such linear notions of time), and this then raises considerable difficulties about how this should be juxtaposed with the experience of bereavement. By putting these different terms together, we could raise a variety of quite disparate issues, as follows:

1   Most specifically, we could be concerned with bereavement that oc-curs during these age groups, and the consequences of such be-reavement for the life experience during those years. This framing of the issue thus uses quite a short time perspective. This is the main area of existing work that specifically links bereavement to young people, who are very largely viewed as 'adolescents' facing particular 'devel-opmental tasks' (see e.g. Balk 1991b; Balk and Corr 1996; Doka 2000).

2   The time trajectory becomes somewhat lengthened if we consider bereavement in the lives of young people, not just by reference to losses they have sustained during the teenage years themselves, but also by reference to deaths they may have encountered during their earlier childhood experiences.

3   An alternative lengthening of the time trajectory occurs if we con-sider bereavement that has occurred during the teenage years speci-fically, but the implications are taken further into the future, in terms of possible outcomes throughout adult life. Studies that take this approach may frame the issues by reference to whether (par-ental) bereavement is seen to have more long-term negative im-plications according to the age at which it occurred, i.e. during early or mid-childhood or during adolescence.

4   The time trajectory may be almost unlimited, however, if the teenage years are viewed as a 'staging post' between 'childhood' and 'adult-hood', framed within the overall life course. In this view, the teenage years *per se* would only be especially relevant if there are seen to be things occurring then that are different from the earlier or later ages.

These different time frames can be represented diagramatically as follows (though with some artificial imposition of cut-off points around age status):

$$- - - - - - (1) - - - - - - - -$$

$$- - - - - - - - - - (2) -$$

____ childhood _____ I ____ youth ____ I _____ adulthood _____

$$- - - - - - - - - - - - - - - - (3) -$$

$$- (4) -$$

The complexity of these issues in terms of the potentially relevant literatures available will be considered further particularly in Chapter 4, where we discuss the quantitative research literatures. For now, we want explicitly to recognize that:

- on the one hand, the conjoining of 'bereavement' and 'young people' can lead to a somewhat arbitrary and artificial slicing of the research literature available;
- on the other hand, we need to keep open a theoretical and empirical space for considering whether the teenage years do indeed raise particular issues for experiences of bereavement.

Most of the literature is framed within the first or fourth time trajectories, in the sense that it either focuses on the teenage years within quite a limited time span, or it only discusses the teenage years in a fairly incidental way. Balk (1995) concludes that we know very little about longer, but ongoing, processes to do with adolescent bereavement (i.e. the third time trajectory above), because studies do not generally follow people up in this way over any period of time (we will discuss those longitudinal studies that do consider bereavement as a longer-term 'risk' factor in a quantitative way in Chapter 4). Balk, for example, suggests that there is evidence of the significance of unresolved grief issues as a factor in students seeking counselling help at universities. Furthermore, where people look back from adulthood to bereavement during childhood (e.g. Holland 2001), it is apparent that grieving can recur at various points in the life course, particularly in relation to key life events (and see the personal accounts discussed in Chapter 3). Similarly, suggestions have been made that a child who may have coped with an earlier bereavement may then experience re/new(ed) grief during adolescence (Furman 1970 cited by Brown 2002). So young people who have been bereaved in childhood might experience further grief issues connected with key life events, such as passing their driving test, getting married, graduating etc. It is also possible that an earlier childhood bereavement might still be relevant to the life experiences of teenagers (i.e. the second time trajectory above), without necessarily being relevant later in life, which would not necessarily 'show up' in the quantitative studies that look at adult outcomes. This raises issues about the point at which 'outcomes' can be said to have occurred (discussed further in Chapter 4).

Besides the empirical complexities of these different time frameworks, however, we also need to note their theoretical implications. While there may be some variability between the first two time trajectories presented above, in terms of when the loss itself occurred, they share a concern with the implications for the life experiences of these age groups as important *in their own right*, with a perspective on the present, rather than viewing them as important only within a longer-term developmental perspective, with a perspective on young people as being in a process of *becoming* something else (James *et al.* 1998). In this regard, the implications of the bereavement experience may be viewed in a fairly short-term time frame. This may be extended, however, if there is an explicit focus on the implications for experiences of 'transition'.

In terms of the third and fourth time trajectories identified, the significance of the teenage years is understood by reference to bereavement experiences for the remainder of the life course overall. In the fourth approach, particularly, where the teenage years are framed as a sort of 'window' in the life course, these years may potentially be considered for the light they shed on the *long-term processes* by which early bereavements may be experienced and mediated during these years, as part of the overall life consequences for individuals concerned.

It will be clear, then, from this discussion, that any literature on 'young people' and 'bereavement' may be framed quite differently with respect to the time perspective involved, with quite different implications for how these literatures may be identified.

We return to issues of time in relation to bereavement experiences in Chapters 3 and 4, but next we consider the theoretical underpinnings to those psychological approaches that do provide a clear focus on issues of bereavement during the teenage years in their own right, using the second time trajectory identified above.

Psychological approaches to bereavement, grief and adolescence

As outlined earlier, psychological approaches to bereavement issues in the teenage years have been based on the perspective of adolescence as a development phase. An early question that was raised within this developmental psychology literature centred on whether children can grieve in the adult understanding of the word, since their cognitive capacities are seen to be immature. Nevertheless, whatever conclusions may be reached about younger children in this regard, the psychological literature concurs that teenagers certainly grieve and have the cognitive maturity to understand death. This, however, points to a key ambiguity in that the ages 10 to 12 are often described as the period at which a 'mature' concept of death is acquired, but often teenagers are shielded from 'adult' experiences of death (Corr and McNeil 1986).

Chronological age and developmental issues are also jointly at stake in discussion regarding whether there is a particular 'worst time' to be significantly bereaved, for example, of a parent. Mack (2001), however, found no effect concerning the age of the child at the time of death of a parent. Overall, Fleming and Balmer (1996: 145) point to a lack of 'solid and consistent findings' in relation to differences of age at time of bereavement within the adolescent years. Nevertheless, empirical studies of the significance of age of bereavement involve complex issues, not only because much depends on which particular 'outcome' or developmental task is being measured, but also because age at time of death is often confounded with time elapsed *since* death.

From the perspective of theories of adolescence, questions continue to be raised as to whether there are particular issues to consider with regard to bereavement at this developmental phase. Raphael (1984) identified adolescence as a key stage when the death of a parent may be seen as problematic. The reason for this is viewed as the additional stress associated with bereavement that can lead to a tension between the need to be protected and regress on the one hand (because of the bereavement), and the expectation of maturity (as a developing adolescent) on the other. The bereavement response of adolescence is therefore theorized as conflictual. A further (socially based) tension may be the perception of taking on more responsibility as a consequence of bereavement, in contrast to being excluded from decision-making within the family (Holland 2001; McNally 2005).

Such psychological approaches to adolescence as a developmental phase elaborate particular tasks around individual development, and physiological changes such as sexuality and aggression. The work of Fleming and colleagues (Fleming and Adolph 1986; Fleming and Balmer 1996) is now widely cited in the psychological and therapeutic literature (e.g. Doka 2000) as providing the most relevant theoretical framework for understanding bereavement and adolescence. In this model adolescence is defined as 11–21, divided into three periods with specific tasks and conflicts. Bereavement is seen as interfering with this 'natural progression'. Adjustment to death, it is argued, will partly reflect the developmental task that was being faced at the time of the death.

Such developmental theories of adolescence point (generally in a very universalistic way) to various issues in relation to bereavement, including:

- *Particular ambivalences concerning relationships.* These may nclude the urge for autonomy etc. – for example, 'the death of a parent creates excruciating anguish for an adolescent ... complicated by tensions over the developmental crisis of dependency versus autonomy that marks adolescent-parent relations' (Balk 1995: 421).
- *Cognitive capacities.* For example, Ross Gray (discussed by Balk 1995) found that there was a clear decline in academic performance among bereaved adolescents under 15, and Balk suggests this may reflect the importance of cognitive development at this age.

- *Identify formation.* For example, as discussed earlier, Balk (1995: 130) centralizes the search for identity, meaning and understanding of self as 'the overarching theme of adolescent personal development'. This is a process that continues throughout life, but he argues that adolescence involves many significant changes that feed into identity formation, such that his own research into adolescence and the implications of bereavement is framed by reference to this central question.
- *Particular risks of psychopathology.* For example, Beratis (1991) discusses adolescence as a period of particular vulnerability to psychopathology (Freud), a period of fluidity and great turmoil.

From a rather different theoretical framework, in a comparison of responses to significant bereavement experiences of younger (twenties) and older (sixties) persons, Barnes *et al.* (1996) found that older people reported more positive emotions and fewer negative emotions than younger interviewees. These researchers suggest that this is linked to a tendency among older people to use 'account-making' and 'confiding' as means of coping (linked in turn to earlier loss experiences), whereas younger interviewees tended to use 'postponing' as a coping strategy.

Hogan and DeSantis (1994) suggest that there have been changes over time in the sorts of psychological *outcomes* that have received attention in adolescent bereavement research, with the 1980s work centred more on psychosocial and cognitive development, while the 1990s saw a shift of interest towards implications for self-concept, grief, personal growth and ongoing attachment. They also discuss a shift from a focus of attention on possible problems of psychopathology, towards risks of social and emotional problems. (This empirical literature is discussed in detail in Chapter 4.)

Besides such different theoretical bases for the *outcomes* considered in research on bereavement and adolescence, the literature is also framed by other notable variations of focus. One such difference concerns the *category of the relationship* with the deceased person – whether a parent, sibling, friend, peer, (unborn) child etc. The bases for such divisions in the literature are rarely made explicit in these studies, but might be assumed to depend on prior theorizing about the significance of different relationships for adolescent development. The death of a parent, for example, may be theorized as particularly significant in the context of tensions concerning the 'developmental crisis' of 'dependency versus autonomy' (Balk 1995: 421; see also Tyson-Rawson 1996). Sibling relationships, on the other hand, may be theorized as particularly significant for identity formation. The absence of such implicit theoretical underpinnings may perhaps be associated with the paucity of work concerning peer bereavement within this psychological framework, although peer group relationships generally have received considerable attention within the sociological literature on youth. One further particular gap that appears when we put these different dimensions of the research foci together is that there appears to be little attention paid at all to situations where a young person may not have any sort of prior relationship with the deceased person, but may nevertheless be significantly affected by the death (e.g. by witnessing a violent death).

Another contour that may be found in the existing psychological literature concerns the *nature of the death itself* – whether anticipated or traumatic, due to suicide or other forms of violence, abortion, infertility etc. The bases for this division may depend on implicit theories about the relevance of time (in the context of anticipated death) (see e.g. Christ 2000) and of post-traumatic stress (in the case of violent deaths) (see e.g. Brent *et al.* 1994; Pfefferbaum *et al.* 1999).

In the process of developing such variable research contours, however, different implications arise concerning how far, and in what ways, we may see dis/continuities between different types of bereavement experience. The ways in which such research parameters are drawn also has the consequence of drawing our attention to certain experiences more than others, such that our knowledge of bereavement in the context of the lives of young people may become quite partial, based on assumptions that are not always explicated.

It is possible, in principle, to develop a 'map' of the literature concerned with these sorts of cross-cutting dimensions, in particular, regarding (1) category of loss, (2) nature of death and (3) outcomes investigated. What is immediately apparent from such an exercise is that the research literature has centred most heavily on bereavement through death of a parent, followed by death of a sibling. Each of these areas now constitutes an extensive research literature in its own right, albeit often quite self-referential and often without being contextualized by reference to what is known about other forms of bereavement. The nature of the death itself is less often used as a basis for defining the focus of research studies, although there is some specialist literature particularly available regarding bereavement through traumatic death, especially suicide, in the context of adolescence (for some examples see Eth and Pynoos 1994; Dyregrov *et al.* 1999; Cerel *et al.* 2000; Pfeffer *et al.* 2000; Raviv *et al.* 2000; Stuber *et al.* 2002).

The variability of outcomes that is considered in research studies in this area is enormous, and is particularly divided between social, educational, physical and mental health factors. What exactly is placed under such headings may itself depend on the ways in which any particular issue is theorized, for example, is delinquency a form of social deviance or an indication of individual behavioural pathology? These complexities in the empirical research literature will be explored in subsequent chapters.

Conclusion

In theorizing 'young people', we find a sharp duality, between psychological work centred on ideas of 'adolescent development' and sociological work centred on 'youth' as a relational social status. It is striking, however, that some common concepts occur across the separate literatures of bereavement and young people, particularly those of 'transition' and 'disruption'. This raises questions as to whether the conjunction of bereavement and youth may be regarded as particularly risky and difficult, since both may involve very significant changes (transitions) and may involve threats to existing social or personal order (disruptions).

But, while we have sought to take a broad overview of theoretical frameworks in this chapter, we also need to stress the cultural limitations of this discussion. In the very different context of a society where violence and early death are pervasive, like Columbia, direct personal experience of death, and a contemplation of one's own death, may be commonplace among young people. The implications of such a different experience can include a return to religion, a selective and creative use of consumer culture, or experiences of early parenthood, as young people actively seek to find ways of living meaningfully in the face of such dangers (Amaya 2002).

Such work draws our attention to the ways in which not only experiences of death, bereavement and grief, but also meanings of what it is to be a child or young person (as discussed earlier in this chapter), have to be considered alongside such particular cultural contexts. Jonker (1997: 165) points out, for example, that within the Muslim faith communities, 'Children are not permitted to attend ... rituals, are discouraged from asking questions and expected to forget the death as soon as possible'. On the other hand, other writers suggest (Young and Papadatou 1997: 199) that 'In traditional cultures ... children ... are exposed to and learn from the same realities as adults – no special arrangements are made to shield or exclude them, as they so often are in the West'. At the same time, children in less affluent cultures or circumstances may well find that the material consequences of the death of the main family breadwinner may emphasize their own importance as members of the labour force and potentially significant contributors to the household income (Strange 2005).

While cultural issues relevant to experiences of bereavement in the context of contemporary multi-cultural Britain have received increasing attention from those professionally concerned with the care of dying and bereaved persons (see e.g. Neuberger 1987; Parkes *et al.* 1997a), Desai and Bevan (2002) point out that 'cultural sensitivity' is not enough as an approach to issues of race in bereavement contexts, and can even increase discrimination through the dangers of stereotyping, failing to attend to the fluidity and disorderliness of culturally patterned everyday experiences (Gunaratnam 1997), and the ways in which cultures may change as minority ethnic groups adapt to their new social contexts (Field *et al.* 1997). In discussing cross-cultural differences, Parkes (2005) suggests that variations can include: the nature of attachments and childrearing practices in the first place; whether there is support for the expression or inhibition of grief; the rituals attending death and mourning; and religious beliefs about death and bereavement. Walter (1999) suggests that a significant source of variation will also occur in terms of whether the bereavement is felt as a loss by groups as well as by a few isolated individuals. Other writers also point to the difficulties of understanding and interpreting experiences of bereavement and expressions of grief across different societies (Scheper-Hughes 1992), and different social groups in particular historical periods (Strange 2005).

Neimeyer (2001) observes that there has, in recent years, been an increasing emphasis on 'local' practices for accommodating losses, and a reduced emphasis on theories of universal processes of grief. In considering such issues, Rosenblatt (2001: 288) suggests that there do appear to be some commonalities across all societies, in the way that 'death seems to be difficult for many people in every culture'. However, drawing on anthropological evidence, he also uses a social constructionist theoretical approach to suggest that cultural differences are very wide-ranging, including, 'cultural understandings of what has been lost with a death, death rituals, cultural constructions of a survivor's ongoing and future relationship with the deceased, and the cultural construction of culturally deviant grieving' (p. 286). At the same time, he stresses the need to understand that, within the context of interactions and relationships shaped by power differences as well as by cultural contexts, 'what follows a death may be as much discussion, interpretation, and social transaction as it is ritual' (p. 295). In this respect, this approach parallels those (mentioned above) who caution against seeing cultural differences as somehow open to orderly categorization and description. Rosenblatt concludes, therefore 'that grieving is malleable, that there is not a simple biological or developmental process that controls and shapes how people grieve a death, how long they grieve, or what meanings they give to the death' (p. 297).

While cultural differences may be highlighted by anthropological and historical evidence, it is psychological perspectives (of bereavement and loss, including adolescent bereavement) that are preponderant within existing, western-based, theoretical literatures concerned with death, dying and bereavement. This is in sharp contrast with the much more limited contribution of sociological perspectives (of the sociohistorical contexts and understandings of death and dying in western societies). This current predominance of psychological theories about bereavement and young people raises questions as to whether this in itself reflects the sequestration of experience in contemporary western societies. Bereavement as such has received little sustained attention from sociologists. Even within the sociology of death and dying, bereavement has rarely featured as an issue except in the context of discussions about mourning rituals and cultural practices. Instead, 'bereavement' *as a concept* is much more firmly rooted in the literatures of counselling, and some aspects of medicine. In these literatures, bereavement is readily understood in relation to various key theoretical and intervention issues, including:

- attachment and loss;
- risk of individual pathology or deviance;
- (ab)normal grief reactions, processes and stages;
- (assessment of) mental health;
- deprivation and multiple disadvantage.

It is these latter frameworks that provide theoretical underpinnings for the great majority of research studies in this area, and it is this empirical work that will be considered in Part 2.

PART 2
Evidence

3 The perspectives of young people

Sue Sharpe, Jane Ribbens McCarthy and Julie Jessop

Introduction

In turning to consider the research evidence available concerning young people's experiences of bereavement, we will start by exploring what we know about the perspectives of young people themselves. However, although the research literature on young people and bereavement has grown significantly over the last two decades, there continues to be a dearth of research which looks specifically at their own perceptions and understandings. And yet such meanings are likely to be a central issue that mediates the impact of any particular bereavement (see Chapter 4).

In this chapter we will first consider the various research approaches that have sought (or potentially could seek) to listen to the perspectives of young people. We will then introduce five new case studies written especially for this project. These are drawn from a major study that has been researching the lives of young people in the UK generally over several years. The case studies are able to present a range of bereavement experiences from young people who spontaneously discussed such issues in the course of the interviews. Finally, we will draw on these case studies, as well as other evidence available, to consider emergent themes from the voices of bereaved young people.

Approaches to qualitative research

It is an increasing trend for young people themselves to be used as respondents in more structured, quantitative research projects (e.g. in the major UK studies of particular cohorts or other samples of the general population). It is particularly striking that Wadsworth (1991) reports, on the basis of the 1946 longitudinal study,[1] that when these people reached age 36, parental

---

[1] These large-scale cohort studies are discussed further in Chapter 4.

death was the single most frequently cited issue by both women and men as something they wished had been different about their lives. But to hear about young people's experiences and understandings in a more open-ended way we need to turn to more qualitative, in-depth studies.

Nevertheless, distinctions between more quantitative/structured approaches, and more qualitative/open-ended approaches are by no means clear-cut (Bryman 2001). Questionnaire/survey-based studies may themselves incorporate aspects that allow us to hear about young people's concerns more directly, while qualitative approaches themselves – as we go on to discuss below – vary a good deal in terms of how exactly they may elicit and – just as importantly – interpret the views of young people.

There has been a general growth in social research that seeks to hear 'the voices' of research participants, often as part of a radical attempt to represent the views and understandings of less powerful groups in society, including work from feminist, post-colonial, queer, and the 'new childhood' studies. This has been associated with much debate about how to theorize what we mean by 'voice', and about the possibilities and limitations of research methodologies that seek to include such voices in public debates and discourses (Ribbens and Edwards 1998). These are difficult issues, to which there are no definitive answers.

In the present context, it is the work from the 'new childhood studies' (see Chapter 1) that is particularly relevant. While this work covers a broad array of perspectives and methodologies, an important element is that it has largely sought to question, deconstruct, or at least sidestep those psychological perspectives that are rooted in a developmental theoretical framework. Instead the aim has been to seek to study and understand the lives of children and young people on their own terms, taking a view of childhood as a phase of life that is socially constructed as much as biologically given, often drawing on sociological or anthropological disciplinary orientations and concepts. Nevertheless, the nature of the research process, and how it is written and presented within academic contexts, is recognized as inevitably invoking an interpretive framework. It is acknowledged that there can be no 'true' rendition of the 'voices' of children or young people: not only may these voices themselves be highly contingent and ambiguous, but the researcher is always part of the context, production, selection and interpretation of such voices.

Again, underlying all these qualitative approaches is the question of whose 'voices' get heard in research studies in the first place. This not only raises issues about which young people in particular are identified for inclusion in any particular research study, but also about the willingness of young people to 'talk about' their lives and experiences, leading to a self-selecting 'bias' in the sample of voices being heard. In this context, it is striking that, even among those children and young people who have spontaneously taken the step to pick up a phone to call ChildLine (the UK anonymous helpline for children), there may be a strong mix of views about whether or not they see talking as helpful: 'Mum died, Dad is too raw to discuss it.' 'Everyone keeps ringing me up. I can't stand it' (callers to Child-Line quoted by Cross 2002: 16).

This raises major methodological issues about how we regard the significance of talk and spoken communication as a source of insight into people's lives. In recent years there has been a general growth of interest in qualitative research methodologies, often used in relation to a variety of 'personal', 'private' or 'family' based issues, but these approaches rely on interviewees being willing and able to talk in depth about their lives and to explain their views and feelings through such talk. This in turn points to features of social change generally in contemporary western societies, with the suggestion that the conditions of high modernity have led to an increasing emphasis on the 'reflexive project of the self' (Giddens 1991). It is thus argued that individuals are expected to be in charge of their own destinies and biographies, with talk and communication constituting central features of such biographies. Furthermore, this emphasis on the construction of a coherent life narrative has also become a feature of some therapeutic approaches, such that this may in itself be understood as indicative of some sort of psychological adjustment to difficult events.

In asking people to participate in in-depth research interviews, then, are researchers themselves contributing to, and drawing on, these wider social changes, such that we are expecting interviewees to become skilled narrators of their own reflexively created biographies (Alldred and Gillies 2002)? And if so, what of those individuals who do not feel able to participate in research using such approaches? Are we in danger of building our research on the views of people who centralize talk in their lives generally, and, furthermore, feel able to use such talk to produce a coherent account of their experiences in an interview setting? This means we have to be very careful about developing any general theories regarding young people's experiences of bereavement on the basis of those who are willing/able to talk about such experiences. This is especially true of any conclusions we may want to draw about the significance of talk and communication in helping bereaved young people.

Varieties of qualitative materials

Bearing all these caveats in mind, it may be helpful for the purposes of the present discussion to distinguish between a variety of more qualitative literatures that may provide us with insights and understandings into the experiences of young people with regard to issues of bereavement. Such qualitative literatures thus potentially comprise at least the following types of work:

1   Autobiographical, anecdotal, practice-based or 'case' materials that are included in 'popular' publications that have been developed as resources for those working directly with bereaved young people. See, for example, Wallbank (1991) and Mallon (1998) for general advice books concerned with children, and Bode (1993) and Levete (1998) for advice books specifically concerned with the teenage years, the latter notably including experiences of young people from a variety of ethnic backgrounds. Examples of autobiographical materials include the books by Abrams (1992) (following the death of her father, the eminent sociologist Philip Abrams), and by Perschy (1997), whose mother died when she was 16. These are generally discussed within a theoretical framework that draws upon established theories of bereavement and grief processes.

2   The work done by ChildLine provides a unique insight into the concerns of a particular selection of young people, namely those who have called in for telephone contact, advice or support. This service is in a unique position in being accessible directly to young people themselves at a time of their choosing. Cross (2002) reports the experiences of child callers to ChildLine (mainly girls in the 11–16 age range) whose reason for phoning has been categorized as primarily concerned with issues of bereavement (a total of 2619, or 1 per cent of total calls made to ChildLine in the years 1998–2000). Videos produced by the Leeds Animation Workshop and also the Childhood Bereavement Network are further examples of resources developed for those working with bereaved young people, which place the 'voices' of young people centre stage (and see also discussion in Chapter 5 for websites for bereaved young people).

3   Individual 'cases' which are included within academic, clinical and/ or professional publications, as a means of exploring and illustrating existing theoretical perspectives (e.g. Balk 1995, 2000; Doka 2000). Some of these materials have been produced within a fairly structured research design, which has nevertheless also incorporated more open-ended questions that are then analysed using a more qualitative approach, for example Worden (1996). Some psychological studies have thus investigated the aftermath of bereavement among adolescents specifically, in quite an open-ended way, and we draw on some of this work in other chapters. Balk (1995) suggests that some of these studies present a generally more optimistic picture of the bereavement experience than other research.

4   Research that is ethnographically framed, which may seek to explore

young people's accounts of bereavement in ways that explicate the salience of bereavement issues in the various contexts of their lives overall, paying careful attention to young people's own use of language, concepts and sets of meanings.

5   Research that is framed by a narrative approach to the understanding of individual interviews, seeking to explore how young people themselves might construct and understand the significance of bereavement experiences in the context of their overall life story.

In relation to the current focus of concern – young people and bereavement – it is very clear that there is far more published material available that falls into the first three qualitative approaches outlined above, and very little that falls into the last two categories. One exception is that of Kenny (1998). As part of a wider study, based in a specific urban locality in the North of England, Kenny held focus groups with 20 young people between the ages of 18 and 23 on their general attitude to death, and posits the view that 'their attitude to death is mainly governed by their attitude to life' (p. 48). The spiritual or existential elements of their views were apparent and many believed in reincarnation. Kenny also obtained retrospective accounts of childhood bereavement from older participants, particularly in relation to wartime deaths and rituals.

Kenny's work is an example of more ethnographically-based work, but this style of research is almost entirely absent in the research literature concerning bereavement and young people. An interesting example, however, in relation to bereavement among adults, is provided by Handsley (2001) who uses a form of autobiographical ethnography to explore family-based events and experiences after the sudden death of a child in the context of an Irish community. Ethnographic work concerned with the care of the dying (e.g. Hockey 1990) has tended to focus primarily on the contexts of death and dying, or on ritual and shared practices of mourning, rather than an analysis of grief and bereavement in daily life.

Besides the possible significant contributions that might be gained from such ethnographies, we discussed earlier, in Chapter 2, the possibilities of more sociological theorizing of grief that would provide a different context for researching young people's perspectives on death and bereavement. We will return to some of these issues in Chapter 6, but one particularly relevant strand here, that in fact traverses some of the familiar disciplinary boundaries, is that of narrative construction, which can be considered as a form of (sociological and social psychological) theory, a research methodology and also a strategy for intervention (Neimeyer 2002).

As a research strategy, narrative approaches are very much rooted in qualitative methodologies, with an emphasis also on the goal of exploring how people themselves understand their lives, and seek to find and develop a sense of meaningfulness from major biographical events (e.g. in the context of health issues more generally – Kleinman 1988). In this respect, then, this approach also resonates with spiritual or existential questions. Narrative research often seeks to elicit life course perspectives and storylines, so that bereavement may then be analysed in terms of, for example, biographical disruptions (Exley and Letherby 2001) or critical moments within the overall narrative (Thomson *et al.* 2002).

Such an approach towards an understanding of individual lives in social contexts has burgeoned in recent years in social research generally, along with a proliferation of debates about how to theorize and interpret such narratives. Seale (1998), for example, argues that bereavement narratives do presume a material reality of death behind the text of the narrative itself. Neimeyer and Anderson (2002 drawing on the work of Angus *et al.*) discuss bereavement narratives as external (accounts of actual events and circumstances); internal (accounts of emotional and experiential responses to events); and reflexive (narratives that seek to 'analyse, interpret and make meaning of an event') (p. 53).

Overall, then, these different qualitative approaches and sources provide variable scope and routes for theorizing and researching young people's understandings of and perspectives on bereavement experiences. It is important to be aware that many of the sources discussed above must be assessed very cautiously as research evidence of how young people generally experience bereavement: while they may provide important insights, we are generally given no information about who exactly these young people might be considered to represent, how they came to be included and on what basis their experiences have been voiced and written up. Krementz (1983), for example, interviewed a number of bereaved young people and wrote them up as case studies, without commentary, using a style that appears to allow the young people to 'speak for themselves'. Nevertheless, Krementz has inevitably shaped the resulting narratives in major ways, through her choice of interviewees, the nature of her involvement with them, and her decisions about how to write up the resulting case studies. These are key issues in enabling us to understand the basis of these written accounts, but none of this information is available, nor is it usually provided in this sort of publication.

Furthermore, while all writing necessarily requires that young people's perspectives be re-framed and re-presented in particular (highly selective) ways, qualitative approaches vary greatly in the extent to which they 'hold open' a space for analysing first order (topical) constructs (Hammersley and Atkinson 1995) and understanding an account as a whole, or instead analyse and present young people's words via pre-existing theoretical frameworks. All of these have their own value, but it is important to be aware of the variability that may occur within the overall umbrella of 'qualitative approaches'.

Young people's narratives of bereavement

There are key methodological and theoretical issues to be considered, then, in relation to the question of whose voices are being heard, and on what basis, in the literature available concerning young people's experiences of bereavement. One crucial element of this concerns whether the young people are being interviewed because they are already known to have been bereaved, which is the basis of almost all the literature discussed above. But such a basis for inclusion is likely to be systematically associated with important differences in the nature of the accounts that may be voiced. There is also an important distinction to be made between those studies that report the perspectives of young people as they are expressed during their teenage years (or very soon thereafter) and those that are based on accounts given by older adults who are looking back, providing retrospective accounts of their teenage experiences.

In these regards, the case studies we present below make a particular contribution to the existing qualitative literatures discussed above, in that:

- these are young people who have *not* been interviewed as part of a study of bereavement as such, but as part of a general study of the lives of young people in contemporary Britain;
- between them they discuss a considerable range of different bereavement experiences, many of which receive scant attention in the existing bereavement literatures;
- they have been repeatedly interviewed on an open-ended, in-depth basis about their life experiences over a period of several years, so that their discussions of bereavement can be set into a holistic context of their lives overall over time;
- their analysis has not been undertaken through a pre-existing theoretical framework concerning processes of bereavement and grief, but through the use of a general narrative approach.

These case studies are derived from the work undertaken by a team of researchers at South Bank University (headed by Professors Janet Holland and Rachel Thomson).[2] In the present context, this work is particularly interesting

---

[2] We are indebted to South Bank University for providing access to these materials. Further details of the studies and associated publications can be found at www.sbu. ac.uk/fhss/ff/. The three studies were funded by the Economic and Social Research Council in their programmes on Childhood (6–16), and Youth, and within the South Bank University Family and Social Capital Research Group, respectively.

as a major source of large-scale, longitudinal qualitative data about the lives of 'ordinary' young people in the contemporary British context. This data set is based on questionnaires and interviews with a total of 1700 young people, some of whom have been followed up in three successive studies over a period of up to seven years (and still ongoing), drawn as community-based samples from schools in a variety of locations across the UK. As part of the analysis of these data sets, the researchers included the issue of whether or not the young people talked spontaneously about bereavement or death as a feature of their lives, and it is thus possible to identify those accounts which include issues of bereavement as discussed by young people themselves. Furthermore, in these accounts, discussion of bereavement was not a focus of the interviews, and so it is contextualized by the ways in which the young people narrated their lives overall, as part of their involvement in the various research projects.

In selecting the case studies for presentation here, young people were identified who had discussed issues of bereavement in their interviews, and we then selected five for in-depth analysis, using the criteria:

- that they would include young people who had not had any particular interventions in connection with their bereavements from relevant services;
- none of them had been identified as particularly 'problematic' young people by any form of statutory body (although Brian did have special needs support during his school life);
- that between them they represented a variety of locations and social experiences in terms of gender and ethnicity;
- that they should span a range of bereavement experiences covering a variety of relationships, and where bereavements were discussed that were more or less central to their accounts, and more or less disruptive of their lives overall.

The five people we chose are:

- Shirleen: a young woman who had experienced a bereavement (of her great grandfather in Jamaica) which featured as a significant part of her life story, but which was not the dominant theme of her narrative.
- Khattab: a young man who discussed several different bereavements in his interviews over the years, including his two grandmothers, and more recently, a much younger woman who was a close family friend, all of which had significant implications for his religious beliefs.
- Maeve: a young woman who encountered several bereavements, including among her close friendship group, which were experienced

as very disruptive at the time, and had implications for her life narrative over the years.

- Brian: a young man whose father died with significant consequences for his life narrative.
- Neville: a young man whose mother died suddenly and traumatically, and whose narrative is dominated by this bereavement.

The interviews from these five individuals were then analysed as narratives by Sue Sharpe,[3] who had not been involved in other aspects of the current literature review, and who therefore had no knowledge of what the existing research evidence has to say about bereavement and young people. Instead, she was given the brief of seeking to immerse herself in the individual accounts, to consider the major themes and events that the young people themselves developed in their interviews. Here we present the resulting case studies, along with some further thoughts about the sorts of themes and puzzles that we have considered as we have engaged with these young people's narratives, as external, internal and reflexive accounts (Neimeyer and Anderson 2002).

Across these various case studies, then, we can gain insights into how a range of bereavements may feature as part of a young person's ongoing construction of their narrative biography and sense of identity. Their bereavement experiences can thus be understood by reference to their particular lives, with regard to the multi-faceted and interwoven layers of personal meanings, family and other close social relationships, cultural contexts and structurally framed resources and constraints that constitute elements of their narratives. It is thus possible to understand the significance of the bereavements discussed by reference to each young person's life narrative overall, providing a particular context of meaning in each case.

Shirleen

Shirleen was interviewed five times between the ages of 13 and 17, the last time when she had moved from school to college to do her A levels. When first interviewed she was living with her mother in a two-bedroom flat. Her mother and father were both originally from Jamaica but were now divorced. She did not see a lot of her father and her half-brother, and explained that she did not get on with her father particularly well.

---

[3] Sue Sharpe is one of the researchers working on the studies at South Bank University. The other core members of the research team are Sheila Henderson, Janet Holland, Sheena McGrellis and Rachel Thomson; Robert Bell, Rebecca Taylor and Tina Grigorio have also been involved with different stages of the project.

But Shirleen and her mother got on really well, and throughout her teenage years she described them as being friends, rather than just being mother and daughter:

> My mum tells me everything what to do, what not to do, where I should be, and I listen to my mum, we're like, we're not like mother and daughter, we're friends . . . she's told me right and wrong from when I was little so that's where I get it from . . . I do talk to mum about everything, boyfriends, everything.

She described how her mother had worked hard as a chef in a restaurant, and then as a catering supervisor for schools. She was always quite strict:

> I was taught about discipline from a young age and I've actually been disciplined quite a lot . . . I think it may be because of my grandparents as well, 'cause if they discipline me I always have to do it, I won't argue back, I would never do that 'cause like they're older and you should respect them.

Her mother always emphasized the value of working at school for her future, and Shirleen had taken that on, it seemed to be a family trait:

> . . . all my family, like my mum pushes me and their mums push them as well so, that's what it's like in my family, you get pushed to do the maximum.

In secondary school, Shirleen spoke of how she always worked hard and in her first years was involved with activities like singing and music, and art and textiles. As well as these, she had been doing tae kwon do (a form of martial art) since she was about 7 years old. By the time she was 14, she had achieved several gold medals and was teaching the younger children. She was one of very few girls who did this well. It was something she really enjoyed, and it seemed to give her more confidence, both in and out of school, adding to her experience of self-discipline and responsibility:

> I'm like, it's made me, I've got a lot more self-confidence, just through doing tae kwon do really 'cause it's made me like speak up more and I think that's what's helped me with school, I got to like to answer questions and things.

It also gave her a sense of having to try even harder as a woman:

> It's more about me being a woman 'cause in there there's lots of men, there's only a couple of girls, there's only one woman who trains there . . .

we know what it's like being in there with all them men and all them boys and I think we do try hard, we do try harder than some of the men . . . it's just that like I will try even harder just to get like my point across and to do what I have to do and like every little thing I do, I put in a hundred percent.

But not so long afterwards, when she was nearly 15, Shirleen left tae kwon do as it had become too tiring and clashed with her schoolwork.

Great emphasis was placed on her family – and she had a large one – and she described them as close:

> When one person's in trouble like someone will always be there and even though sometimes it is kind of a having to help, bend over backwards to help, you know they're your family at the end of the day and they'll be there for you in the same kind of situation . . . I'm close to my family, I really am close, if I don't see them for a long time I start to moon about the house, and I have to see them the next day, I'm close to my cousins, my nan, everybody.

Shirleen identified that it was when she was about 12 or 13 that a family illness and death – her great grandfather in Jamaica – had made her think more about herself and life in general:

> I think there's not really been a particular time where something's changed me, but some things that happen, like small things, have made me like who I am, but they haven't been like serious major things, I think I've been more, well my great grandfather died, it was about a couple of years ago and . . . like I knew him but like I went to Jamaica so I could get to know him more, but when he died I think it made me realize that I can't waste the time and seeing that the years are going by so quickly, I don't really have time, I feel like they're just slipping from underneath me sometimes, like a day will come and then the next day is gone.

And it made her even more of a 'family person':

> I went to see him but I think that I could have got to know him a little bit more . . . since then I've like stayed around my family a bit more, more of a family person, that's probably what's made me so close to my family. My grandad's over here, it's not that far so I go down and see my nan and grandad every week . . . I just like to spend time with my grandparents more, since my great grandad died, 'cause I feel like, because they're older, like my grandad's quite ill and so is my nan as well, so I spend more time with them 'cause like sometime they could be gone so I try and spend as much time with them as I can.

In terms of a future career, at 13 Shirleen wasn't sure what to do but she thought maybe art and textiles, or even music. A year later this had changed – she was thinking about being a lawyer, an ambition that would stay with her throughout her subsequent interviews.

At 15 and in her GCSE year she was working really hard, with pressure from her mother and her own strong self-motivation. She was still close to her mother, and they talked quite a lot, but her mother was working nights and slept in the day and was generally very tired. She was against her daughter getting a part-time job because it would impede her schoolwork, so she gave her any money she needed.

Shirleen always felt that she was more mature than the other people in her year. By her own account she was an independent and determined person and wanted to be in control of where her life was going. She also felt that it was not going to be easy to achieve her law ambitions because she was black. Work experience at a law chambers increased this awareness, as the people working there (apart from the clerks) were mainly white and male, but it also increased her determination:

> I think that's what motivates me actually, because you don't see much young black women doing what I'm doing, and I don't see it really, so I think that's what makes me more determined to get where I want to be really. And just to try and keep a sense of self-awareness, just to think of myself, so I identify with what I am really because I know I'm a woman and I know I'm black. So it's just trying to be the best that I can be really and not letting anyone hold me back ... but if I know that I've got the drive and I've got the education to back it up, then I know that whether I'm female I will try and do everything that I want to do and really I'm not gonna let anyone stop me really.

At the age of 17 Shirleen was well into her course at college, where she had met her present boyfriend, Ben, who was 19 and from Nigeria. This relationship seemed to have become quite serious: Shirleen joked they were 'joined at the hip', and it had become a sexual relationship (her first). Her mother approved, as he was a serious student doing similar courses, and in fact they competed against each other, which pushed them both to work even harder. She was taking four A levels, and hoping to go to university the following year to take a law degree. Her life was very full since she now looked after her arthritic nan after college, but she managed to see Ben a lot within this regime. She felt that she had changed a bit in the last year or two and was feeling more 'grown up':

> I think I've got more of a sense of direction, I know what I'm doing, my plans for the future and everything, and now I've got more to consider with Ben and everything, it's like I've got more consideration. I think I've become more considerate about other people's feeling as well.

She had some ideas about the future, such as returning to Jamaica to work, where she hoped her grandparents and mother would also end up:

> I would like to practice law in Jamaica – I don't know what the legal system is like out there but I would like to make a difference, if that doesn't sound too corny or whatever. I would like to practise law here for a reasonable amount of time but I feel I would like to end up in Jamaica regardless.

Because of all her college work, and spending time with her nan, her relationship with her mother, although still close, had changed slightly as well, as she commented: 'I don't really see her much any more, we do have the odd girlie chat sometimes'. But nevertheless, it was her mother who she felt had been a key person in her life:

> She's really pushed me to make me do everything that needs to get done. But like she doesn't ... she balances it up so she doesn't push me too much ... And, she only makes me do things that she knows I will benefit from in the future. And, like, she's just been making me basically knuckle down to my exams the same way that she made me keep at tae kwon do. And she's basically made me stay on track and keep on doing the things I've been doing. She is, like, she's my number one role model. Next to my nan.

It seems that it was her great grandfather's death years ago that helped to make Shirleen realize that she needed to get on and do things with her life, together with her mother's strict encouragement. But at this stage, she was also beginning to feel that there was in fact more time to do things:

> I feel like I've still got a lot to learn and there's still a lot of things that I don't know that I wanna know, that's what my mum says sometimes, I'm a bit too eager [laughs] and to learn everything as soon as possible but now I know that I've got more time than like I thought I had so I can just really kick back for a couple of years and you know, I still got all my life to grow up and do what I wanna do.

Commentary

In terms of this textual analysis, then, we can discern a number of key themes that help to frame the narratives that Shirleen develops through the various interviews. The two central – and closely interwoven – themes would appear to be those of family, and of her mother in particular. Family seems to be the mainstay of Shirleen's life, but it is presented in terms of both breaks (e.g with her father and brother) and continuities (e.g. with family traits over generations). Gender is also central to Shirleen's account, and her mum features as the key person in the earlier interviews, with her nan becoming more central in the later interviews. In this context of key maternal figures, Shirleen describes her life as having been disciplined and pushed in certain directions. This 'pushiness', however, is also 'owned' by Shirleen as time goes on, and she comes to describe herself as a confident, responsible and ambitious person, with the determination to succeed in her chosen goals despite the disadvantages that she perceives from being black and a woman, and these identities are further important themes that are explicated over the interviews. While friendships, peers and boyfriends also feature in Shirleen's accounts, these do not constitute the central figures in the ways that her mum and nan are presented.

It is in this overall context that we hear of the death of her great grandfather in Jamaica, which is discussed at various points in these interviews over the years. We can thus understand the significance of this death in terms of her quest to understand her family history and its links with Jamaica, and thus a key feature of her identity as a black person in a situation of migration and diaspora. The death is also discussed very explicitly in relation to Shirleen's existential perspective on time in the overall life trajectory, as she describes this death as having focused her mind on what her life is about, increasing her sense of determination. Nevertheless, it is also apparent that the meaning of the death is not static, and is reconsidered as Shirleen's own life moves along, leaving us with a puzzle in relation to the complex and rather contradictory views that Shirleen expressed in her last interview, about how far she still views life as needing to be lived in a hurry.

Khattab

Khattab has been interviewed five times between the ages of 15 and 21, spanning the years of his GCSEs, A levels and university. His family come from Pakistan. When first interviewed he was living in a city in the South of England with his mother, stepfather, younger sister and small half-sister. He considered that he had had a 'tough childhood' because his parents split up when he was about 7 and his mother married again. His biological father also remarried and had more children, giving Khattab several more half-sisters, although they did not see each other very much. He felt that he had a reasonable relationship with his stepfather, as long as his stepfather did not try to take his father's place: 'He's alright, so long as he takes care of my mum and the house, you know what I mean, I've got respect for him'.

At age 15, Khattab had a passion for football. Although he was already playing for a semi-professional club, it was his dream to become a professional and eventually return to Pakistan and start a football team there. His family supported him in his footballing aspirations, but he described how his mother was keen for him not to neglect his education:

Mum knows I'm very serious about my football but she also wants my education to be up there . . . That's the thing though, there's a lot of Asian footballers out there, but I've never seen one at professional level yet. So hopefully, my goal is to be the first Asian in the Premiership.

Khattab was very excited at his first interview because he had a forthcoming trial with a professional football club and he was determined to do well, especially because some years earlier he had been trialled by the same club but it had not come to anything. In the event, once again he did not make the team. He told of his intense disappointment, but he continued undaunted, and determined to continue to try to get himself spotted for a professional team:

I'm not going to give up. I'm not going to put my head down and go, 'Oh I'm not going to be a footballer'. That's the thing about me, I never give up. I never want to give up.

He did however succeed in getting nine A–C grades in his GCSEs, which pleased both himself and his mother: 'My main worry was to please my mum. Which I did'. The next thing was A levels and he felt that he was being sensible enough to continue to pursue his education although still desperate for a career as a professional footballer.

He described his family, which was Muslim, as religious with strong beliefs. Unlike many other young people of his age, he did not have much time for social life, spending most of his spare time training or playing football. Because of keeping fit, he did not smoke or drink and said that he certainly did not think about drugs. As a Muslim he was not in any case supposed to drink alcohol:

So in a way there is a link between my football and my religion because the football keeps me off the alcohol, keeps me off the cigarettes and alcohol is a sin to drink in my religion. Also it keeps me off the women . . .

On Saturdays he worked long hours on a market stall to earn a bit of money. He had not made girlfriends a priority, but he definitely wanted to get married one day. There was no arranged marriage in his family, but he knew that he would have to marry a Muslim girl. His mother had already talked to him about marriage when he was about 15:

What she wants me to do first, she wants me to go and take a trip to Pakistan, with me and my mate, have a look around . . . Said, 'If it doesn't work there, come back to England, look for a girl'. Look for a Muslim of course. And she said, 'Erm, if you like her, I'll go and talk to the parents, if they say yeah, you two go out with each for about a year or two, or one year, and then see how it goes from there'.

Khattab discussed his first encounters with death in his family during his first interview when he was talking about the older people in his family. Firstly there was his grandmother (his mother's mother) who had become ill and died in Pakistan some months earlier. His mother went over there but he was unable to go because of his exams. He was quite upset about this and it made him think about people dying, such as his own mother:

> Hope not, but your mum's going to get old one day and the same thing is going to happen. That made me wake up a bit ... some people say religion makes it more easy but I don't think it does. Some people say it was time for her to go to God and all that. It probably was. It was probably time for her. They're old now, my [other] grandma is coming on 80 that's a good age. So, I don't know.

It prompted him to talk to his mother about death and religion:

> Like I asked my mum what that was about, she told me that the thing is when you go to bury the body it's said religiously, that once you turn around there's death angels there. You know like you've got death, like death angels there who pray or something, then they will throw something at you that will make your heart at rest.

In the second interview Khattab described how his other grandmother in England (his paternal grandmother) had since become ill and died. This was even more upsetting for him, as he went to the hospital and saw her afterwards:

> I actually went to the hospital and I saw her face, I mean it was a dead body there and I just saw her face just like, y'know, the mouth was open like she was in pain or something, I just saw her body and I just started crying ... I was upset, I was distressed, I was like I can't believe she was gone ... so I've got no grandparents left.

As if that was not enough, his biological father had a heart attack when he was in Pakistan, and although they were not close, he was extremely concerned that he was going to lose his dad as well. In the event, his father recovered.

At 17, and after many efforts to get football scouts to watch his game, Khattab had still not managed to get selected for a professional team. He was approaching his A level exams and needed to make a decision about what to do next. Reluctantly recognizing that football was still just out of reach, he applied for university. He chose, and was accepted by, a university that was not too far away from his home, so he could return at weekends. He could then continue to play in his team, carry on with his weekend job, and see his family.

By the age of 19, Khattab had passed his exams and gone off to university to study economics. He enjoyed life there, describing it as 'brilliant'. He met new friends, although he said he preferred the old ones: 'Old is gold', he commented. At this time, his aspirations and dreams about football had begun to fade and he was reassessing his values:

> I used to think about, yeah, be a footballer, have all this money, you know and just do something you love, whatever, just follow your heart, but then as soon as I went to uni and I met some of these people I realized that's just you know . . . that's not it, that's not it.

He also realized that he did not want to lose his educational opportunities:

> I don't want to sacrifice my education and find out I can't be a proper footballer . . . I can't afford to lose that but with the football it's like I want it, but it's like the football doesn't want me, so it's really upsetting sometimes.

With his football career disappearing over the horizon, it was becoming Khattab's wish to settle down and have a family in the not too distant future. Although he still had not really had a girlfriend, he had met a young woman who he said he hoped might be his wife one day when he was ready to marry, but because of their shared religion they could not date like other young people.

As well as disappointment with the outcome of his football aspirations, Khattab described how his life had been totally shaken up by the tragic death, from cancer, of the wife of a close friend of his family. This friend was only eight years older than Khattab, and his wife was only 26. Her death at such a young age had a serious impact on his views on life and on his religion:

> I was praying five times a day, I was keeping up, I was doing it because I realized that life's too short. This lady she's only 26 and she's gone. She left two kids behind, so you know it hit me, especially when my grandma passed away and what happened to my dad, I understand that you know, life's too short . . . This death really hit me though, 'cos this was the first death that I came across where the person was only like eight years older than me, it hit me.

He started going to Islamic discussions at university to find out more about religion:

> I started realizing that at the end of the day I've got to, you know, as much as I'm trying to hide it now you know, there is a God and I've got to worship Him so at the end of the day 'cos, I'll leave this life. All this thing about money, wife, child, it's not going to mean nothing if I don't live to see whatever, I don't know whether I'll live to see tomorrow, I don't know when I'll die you know, death doesn't need an invitation does it?

He talked to his mother about his thoughts and feelings. She had been con-cerned about aspects of his increased religious involvement and his need to pray five times a day. She told him, 'It's good to pray, it's good to remember God, but don't forget your life'. He felt that, in many ways, he was questioning life and death, and it was making him much more conscious of the importance of being a Muslim:

> I want to succeed in football, and I want to succeed in education, I want to succeed in life, you know and I want to succeed as a Muslim, that's something else, it's one extra thing but I want to succeed in it. I used to say to myself, I'll look into God when I'm older and I see these people now yeah, they're about 60 or whatever, you know they're old and now they're looking into God and I think it's a bit too late for that 'cos, I mean only God knows but, this lady died at the age of 26. I can't wait until I'm that old, I don't know when I'll die, so that's the only thing, I don't know when death is going to come to me so I've got to prepare for it, try to prepare for death.

His religion, being a Muslim, was still the most important thing in his life, next to his family, and football. At his last interview after achieving his degree, Khattab spoke of how he had always wanted to go on the pilgrimage to Mecca ('Hajj') and planned to go in the next year or so. The experiences of death so far in his life had moved him to question his existence, and towards a deeper involvement in the demands and beliefs of Islam:

> It might sound a bit funny but I think more about, think more about afterlife, now. It sounds a bit crazy but ... I mean I take life one day at a time, how it comes you know. I know I'm going to grow old, I just see myself in the future like you know, I just want a good job, I want to be able to take care of my family, I want to be a good Muslim at the end of the day.

In this context, despite still being anxious to marry, he had renounced social contact with the women he already knew here. Then in his last communication, aged 22, Khattab described how, on a visit to Pakistan, he had met and married a young Muslim woman who was doing a university degree, and was about to bring her back to England and his family home.

Commentary

The two major themes of Khattab's various interviews would seem to be his relationship with his mother and 'success', with his concern to please his mother being an important element of his drive for success. But the focus of the theme of 'success', and the meaning it has for him, varies over time.

Football remains an abiding passion over the years, but it becomes a source of disappointment and upset. At the same time, he appears to rethink its significance as a route to success in terms of fame and money. In these regards, both education and his plans for marriage and family life receive greater priority as time goes on.

But success also gets rethought as a result of his experiences of death and bereavement. Firstly the deaths of his grandmothers, and the possible death of his father, both lead him to consider that his own mother will one day die. But it is particularly the death of his 'uncle's' wife, as someone close to him in age, which has a major impact on his own approach to life, and particularly intensifies his interest in religion. This leads him to ponder the idea that life is short and death is unpredictable, so that he starts to prioritize concerns about life after death alongside concerns about life in this world. At the same time, his religion is also discussed in terms of another area of life where he wants to strive to do well, in order to achieve 'success' as a Muslim, with relevance perhaps both to life in this world and the next.

Maeve

When first interviewed, Maeve was 15 and lived with her parents and older sister in Northern Ireland. She has subsequently been interviewed on four more occasions, most recently at university, aged 19. At the first interview, she appeared to be a sociable young woman, who wanted to combine schoolwork with having good fun. Her older sister had done well and, at the time of the first interview, was moving to England to do a university degree.

Nearly a year later, and now 16, Maeve reflected on how she missed her sister but felt she had had to develop a new relationship with her parents as the only child at home. She was taking 11 GCSEs and thought that she might like a career in medicine. She described how she had quite a large circle of friends, and other activities, but she seemed to be able to juggle her various social, cultural and school worlds. She had a boyfriend who was part of her friendship circle. Her three closest friends also had boyfriends and she was finding this all a bit 'couply'. Friends were very important to her:

> ... me and Charlie, we're both friends in the same friendship group, we don't be all couply, you know, whenever we're all together, it's just like a good laugh, have a bit of craic with all of our friends like ... You've got to be careful, you know what I mean ... friends always come first like.

When interviewed the following year, now aged 17 and a half, Maeve had done really well in her GCSEs. She was doing her A levels and enjoying more freedom and responsibility from the teachers at school, as well as at home. Moving into the A level year was a significant stage for her, but more significant had been the deaths of her grandfather, and a girlfriend, which came quite close together: 'Recently, in the past couple of months, a lot of bad stuff has happened . . . A lot of death'.

Her grandfather had been ill for the previous seven years, and was in residential care. At his funeral, Maeve was surprised to find that she did not cry, but she did acknowledge that she was not greatly upset by his death and commented that it 'was really a good thing because he had been sick for ages'.

The funeral brought the family together in a way that made an impression on Maeve and gave her a closer sense of her family heritage and identity on her father's side:

> All the relations came up and all, so people I didn't really know had come up . . . I actually liked all that side of my family that I had hardly ever met before, you know what I mean. Like, I had met my Great Aunt and like, I like her, she came up and stayed with us and all, and like she's like the only one left in their family . . . but like my granny's family I didn't know at all, and I met them all.

At this time she was still with her boyfriend although they had an agreement to part when they each went to university. Their relationship had become very close and 'nearly sexual'. Her friendship circle had expanded but she was still very much involved with her close friends. She was learning to drive, and had a part-time job in a shop, giving her a financial independence that she liked.

Life seemed to get back to normal after the funeral but then came another death, this one very different and totally unexpected. It was a tragic accident involving Brid, the girlfriend of Maeve's good friend Owen, who died when she was driving with her father and sister and they hit a patch of black ice:

> It was really hazy, nobody knew what exactly happened. Her sister and her daddy were sitting in the front seat, and they were unmarked like. It was just so weird the way she died because it was like fate or something . . . She doesn't like getting into her own car without wearing a seat-belt, and she didn't have one on . . . Like, it's kind of hard to know. And it's so weird, this is the weird thing, it wasn't that she just died. The night before she had a dream that she was at her own funeral in a church and all. Really really weird . . . It was such a freak like, such a freak accident . . . it really, really upset me.

She and her friends went to the wake, and to the funeral:

> I went for the funeral and I hadn't done any work since I had heard, you know, you just couldn't concentrate, so my biology was a disaster because of it. I didn't care like . . . that evening Owen and his daddy and all, all of us were sitting in a bar near his house and we all sat down there, it was

> really really sad but it was dead good, everyone was sitting about and his mummy and daddy were buying us all drinks and everyone was just talking about it and all.

Brid's death had a great impact on Maeve and her friends:

> Everybody is still in a big group, but recently, like since Brid died, nobody has really been in the form for going out, going out for big nights out or anything. And we have been spending a lot of our time together since then as well, then I think it kind of made everybody realize what is important like.

Both deaths were significant for Maeve, but her friend's put the other in perspective: '... it's like old people dying it's not bad, compared to someone who's 18'.

During the next year she moved with her family to a new house some way away, but she still managed to meet up with her friends. Now 18, she was head girl, taking three A levels and hoping to go to university to study medicine.

But this year was tragically affected by yet another death in her friendship group. Describing the period after Brid died as a 'limbo period', she observed:

> ... that was when we thought nothing could get any worse, and do you know, Brid's boyfriend Owen we were all friendly with, he committed suicide about two months after she died ... I mean obviously he was grieving for Brid who he really loved and everything but he didn't give any indications, do you know what I mean?

They were all shocked by his death:

> We went to Owen's house then, the whole gang of us didn't leave each other for like three days, we were just always together and did everything together it was really strange ... God it was terrible. It really changed everyone like. It was his anniversary a couple of weeks ago.

She and her friends found this death very difficult:

> For the whole week we didn't stop crying. We were talking about it afterwards, we rarely talk about it now, for the whole week it was like a steady run of tears of all of us. Didn't know what else to do really. Didn't want to believe it. Still can't sometimes ... at the start everyone was really angry like if he had waited even a month an extra month he would have seen that it wasn't so bad. That he could live without her and he was just too grief stricken he could not see ... and he's gone now and we're still left trying to understand ...

Maeve reflected on how she and others coped and the changes it brought to their relationships, including her own break-up with her boyfriend, because, she said, he became too dependent on her at a time when she needed support herself over the death of her friend:

> I think we overall coped well considering, like it's not something that is supposed to happen whenever you are 18 . . . We had Cruse bereavement people in school and everything talking to us and stuff . . . at the time we were all really, really close to basically all Owen's friends . . . but after that the fellas really, really bonded and excluded us. I think they did it on purpose and then I broke up with Charlie and then in the summer Claire broke up with Sean so we don't really hang around with them any more. That was a big change that came about as a result of his death.

As well as individually, the death had brought other changes to the group of friends as a whole:

> I've got more serious, we all have, just got more serious and less light-hearted, think about things more, more kind of pensive about stuff and plus we don't have any, we hardly ever have, stupid fights or anything or dramas. We used to be the most dramatic group of friends, everything was like panic and we're not like that any more . . . I think it definitely changed us all, it has made us stronger, you can't go through something like that and not change. Especially at a time when everything is chan-ging, when you're 17 a year's a long time . . . It seemed everybody was dying last year. On New Year's Eve, it was like thank God year 2000's over.

And it had put things into perspective:

> I think I'm cold-hearted sometimes as well because old people dying doesn't make me sad at all any more, like Cait's granny I'm like, oh that's terrible, but it doesn't get to me at all because I kind of see it as old people are supposed to die, you are supposed to die whenever you're 75 or 80, it's natural, it's not natural around [that young age].

By the time she was interviewed the following year, aged 19 and a half, Maeve had achieved her aims, and was at university studying medicine, where she'd met a group of friends which felt very secure. Her sister was now living in London, they were still close and she had been there to visit. She kept in touch with her old friends, but it was harder as they were all in different places. But she thought they were still all very close and they always would be. Her parents had missed her at first, and when she came back home for a visit, her mother told her she had changed: 'I think I'm more comfortable with myself, more relaxed I suppose'. Maeve felt she had grown up even more and was more of an equal. She was happy being free and single, not looking for a relationship, and planning her summer holidays.

But death was still to impinge on her indirectly in the form of the brother of her university friend, Hannah, who was killed in a car accident. Hannah had rung her in the middle of the night to tell her what had happened, as she thought Maeve's previous experiences with friends dying made her an appropriate person to ring for advice and support:

> There was no point in saying it but it will get better eventually, it's too early to say that now . . . she felt she had to talk to me or whatever so that's grand, but maybe later on after everything calmed down a bit. I said 'no problem'. A lot of what we do, me and Hannah, our friendship is like, we actually sit and talk . . . I used to sit and listen to her talk about her family you know which is the worst about it, she loved talking about her family all the time so I knew, I feel as if I know them all.

Reflecting on the effects of her experiences, Maeve commented:

> It makes you tougher in a good way but I suppose depending what happens to people, you don't want to go too tough, but it does give you a bit of an exterior.

She likened this process to that experienced by her friend Christina, whose parents had split up when she was young:

> . . . there was this whole mummy, daddy thing, fighting or whatever for years and years and years and that kind of made her tough. Nearly everybody has something, even no matter how small it is. Owen and Brid was mine.

At this point in her life, Maeve was quite clear about her plans for the future, which involved combining travel with qualifying as a doctor before she settled down. Her experiences of death across the life span seemed to have had a clear impact on her attitudes to life, as reflected in many of her observations above, on her family relationships, friendships, and the tragedy of losing lives so young. Asked in the last interview how she may have changed over the years since the beginning of this project she replied:

> God, so much! What age was I – 14 – just growing up, you didn't have a clue anyway at that age like. You think you do but you don't really have a grip on reality. You aren't experienced enough. It's the case now even. Give me a couple of years of life, I'll be an expert.

Commentary

Maeve appears from this narrative analysis to be a very competent young woman, who makes long-term plans for her future which she is able to put into effect. At the same time, she wants a balance in her life, and enjoys the *craic*. Key themes through all her interviews are her friendship groups, with her family constituting a less prominent but still key source of valued support in the background. Increasing independence through the process of 'growing up' is also an important theme. The recurrent deaths that have happened to those around her, at a time when change is a particular feature of the expected life course anyway, are described as having made her 'tougher' and less of a 'softie'. This is not seen as altogether negative, and she regards the bereavements as having given her and her friends a greater sense of 'what's important'. She makes a very clear distinction between the deaths of older and younger people, with the latter seen as having an impact that the deaths of older people don't. It is also apparent, with each bereavement among her friends, how she is striving to make sense of the actual deaths as these have occurred under varying and traumatic circumstances. At the same time, she also sees some continuity between these experiences of bereavement and the situation of her friend whose parents divorced after some years of acrimony. Since she feels that 'Nearly everybody has something' to deal with in their lives, she seems to have been able to incorporate these bereavements into her life experience, despite their devastating impact at the time.

Brian

Brian, who came from a rural part of the East of England, was interviewed four times, between the ages of 15 and 19, by which time he was at college.

Brian had wanted to be an astronaut, but was also very fond of nature and thought forestry would be an alternative career. He and his family – his parents and his brother, who was five years older – had lived in the same house in this country community for most of his life. It felt very secure and safe and he saw life as good. However, the area was not very near his school, and he and a couple of others had to go by taxi. School was less of a safe place. He had a physical problem with coordination, and some learning difficulties (although he went on to take GCSEs), and was assigned a support worker. He tended to be bullied and was in a mixture of ordinary and special needs classes. His family was very important in supporting him in these situations:

> I've had a pretty good life, it's been pretty good . . . and my mum and dad have always been there, when I've been bullied, they've helped me, like just been there for me . . . last time I was bullied was about two weeks ago, my mum helped me through it.

The interviewer involved with Brian commented that he was a young man who always seemed younger than his age and somewhat naïve, and, indeed, he described himself as 'immature, with a daft side' and 'a prankster'. At 15 he did not have a network of friends, but he had a special friend in school at this time called Lisa. Theirs was a relationship contained within school, and kept discreetly secret there because of teasing from others, though they also talked on the telephone, and he thought of her as his 'girlfriend'. But he and Lisa did not go out together, and he spent much of his time at home, watching TV or videos.

During the previous year, Brian's father had become ill and had developed cancer in his lung, which was treated but it recurred six months later. After several weeks it moved to his brain and he died. Talking about this in the interview a couple of months after the funeral, it was clear that this had shattered the security of Brian's life. As his father got increasingly frail he had done his best to help his mother look after him, and now he was concerned with how he could help his mother to cope:

> My mum says just be your normal charming self and help us through it. My mum said she can never be sad when I'm around, 'cause I helped us through it and also helped my dad when he was very poorly, I had to lift him up, mum said that's a great help.

Brian had taken a couple of weeks off school when his father died, and when he returned the people there were quite supportive. Lisa in particular helped and they used to have long talks on the phone in the evenings. He had also talked a bit to his support worker about it.

He described himself as a kind and caring son, and was very attached to his father. He described the special things they had shared, particularly the 'magical Christmases' when decorating the Christmas tree, and he anticipated this would be a hard loss to face when the next Christmas came along:

> I've got all sorts of memories of dad really. Done a lot of good things, made every single Christmas magical … yeah and so did my mum. It's gonna be sad but we're gonna try and make it happy but it's not gonna be the same really without him. It's gonna be hard though 'cause every year me and dad used to put the lights on the tree, every year, so this year it's just gonna be down to me and my brother, and my mum.

A year later, at the second interview, aged 16, he recalled this first Christmas:

> … life's been going alright, been feeling a bit sad now and then … but the hardest part was at Christmas, Christmas Day morning, mum said once we got the meal over Christmas Day, it's alright, but it was in the morning like opening the presents, and I missed him putting the lights up on the tree … it weren't the same … my brother did the lights and I was just hanging stuff up.

At this time, Brian was still at school and contemplating GCSE exams with his father in mind:

> Probably gonna get on with the exams okay, another thing, dad's looking over and dad would want me to do well. That's what I think anyway.

He spoke of how he had grown taller and bigger, but otherwise saw himself as being much the same. His mother had gone back to work as a school mentor/support worker, which made life feel a bit more back to normal. But there had been more illness in his life in that his grandfather had developed bowel cancer. Brian's reaction had been: 'No, don't tell me, not again!' But it turned out not to be fatal.

However, there had been another loss in his life at this time – Lisa. In his role as a caring friend, he had become concerned that she was losing a lot of weight, and had mentioned it to a teacher, as he was afraid she might be anorexic. When she found out she was furious and 'dumped him'. They were no longer speaking, and although clearly hurt by this, he commented, 'I'm a bit sad but it's her loss, ain't it?' He thought this was final, and in his view: 'the cracks are too big to be repaired, the forest has burnt'. He described having other friends at school, mainly younger girls, and said they were supportive and sympathetic, but he still missed Lisa. They were asking him out, but he refused, saying he wasn't ready yet.

He had more or less given up his dream to be an astronaut and was focusing on something more down to earth, like gardening. He definitely wanted a practical job, preferably outside, and he had done some gardening as work experience and enjoyed it. At this time he was not making plans: 'gonna plan every day as it comes'.

Although there was a sense of continuity in Brian's life through his home and family, losing Lisa's friendship had made a dent in this, and his father's tragic death was still very present in his mind:

> Sit there and think and it just makes me feel sad. Sometimes you think about it when you're sad but sometimes you think about it when you're happy, 'cause you remember all the good memories with him.

Brian missed his father a lot, and commented: 'the person close to you would be your dad, your best friend'. In comforting him, people tried to point out some positive things:

> . . . in a way people tell me that I've been lucky 'cause I had a dad who loved me, didn't beat me up, he cared for me and Jeff, and people said, in a way Brian, you're lucky, you had your dad with you for the first 15 years of your life.

His brother had taken over as 'man of the house', doing odd jobs and driving them around. They had got closer in some ways since their dad died, but Brian thought he had become 'too bossy'. But he still thought that he was lucky in that 'I've got a great mum, and a great brother.'

Another year on in his life was to see two more deaths – his grandmother and his father's best friend. At this point, aged 17, he spoke of himself as being 'unlucky' because there was so much death in his life. He still thought about his father's death, and wondered what life would have been like if his father had still been around for him:

> Yeah, still replay it back in my mind, even now, nearly two years ago, wonder what would happen if . . . it's like wouldn't have got the cancer, would he still have been here now, often think that, I think would he be here now?

But one good thing had happened – he and Lisa were friends again, although it was not close like before.

Brian was now taking a horticultural course at college to do gardening, together with maths and IT (he liked computers), with a view to maybe going into forestry. It had been a relief to leave the bullying behind (mainly involving 'calling' his mother or father). He was enjoying being treated as more grown up at college, although for his age he still seemed relatively immature to the interviewer. He said that college had proved easier than he had thought it would be, and a lot more friendly than school. He had never thought he would be able to go to college because of his special needs, so getting a place had been an important event in his life:

> I thought I'd never go college 'cause they know I'm not very good, my coordination's not very good, go to special school . . . went mainstream primary, went to secondary and mum thought I won't get into college and I got in and done alright, so mum's quite proud.

A couple of years later, at 19, college had unfortunately not worked out quite as well as Brian had hoped, and he had taken a year off horticultural studies to take a course in independent skills. His brother had moved out to live with his girlfriend, so it was now just him and his mother at home, and she remained his abiding concern:

> I do have worries for the future, like my mum getting lonely, things like that. Most concerned about my mum a lot. I mean I got my brother but . . . it's my mum that hardly goes out, I get worried sometimes.

Commentary

When Brian was younger he did not seem to the interviewer to have much of a grasp on reality, although he had certainly taken in the reality of his father's death. And he appeared to have no real sense of the long term, and still has little of this. Without the presence of his brother, his narrative places himself now as the man in his mother's life, but while wanting to care for her he is still strongly dependent on her, and looks to her for many things. He could not see his life as being far away from the home and community he has always known. If his father had been there, he suggests, life might have been different, in terms of support for both himself and his mother, and he would still have him as his 'best friend'. Nevertheless, the family had retained some continuity despite the devastation and disruption of losing such a crucial family member (though Brian himself does not discuss it in quite these terms).

Recurrent themes in Brian's interviews concerned issues to do with being 'lucky' or 'unlucky', about bullying, and being different, or mainstream educationally. Some of these themes remain as puzzles, such as the extent and nature of the bullying, which may, perhaps, have been 'played down' in Brian's interviews. As the years passed between the interviews, Brian's accounts shifted from positive accounts of his lucky life, to more apprehensive narratives of a life in which risks had become more apparent. The death of his father was a major event in his life and, although his life did not appear to have taken too much of a turn for the worse as a result, his distress and regret clearly went deep and continued over the years of the interviews. Combined with other losses and deaths of important people around him, Brian would appear to be potentially at risk in terms of his own need for support in the years to come. Nevertheless, his own major concern was with the needs of his mother: it seems that Brian worried about her as much as – perhaps – she might worry about him. A further person in this equation is his brother, who remains an unknown quantity with regard to the future needs of both Brian and his mother.

Neville

Neville has been interviewed five times altogether. His first 'interview' was a 'one-man' focus group, aged 17, when he was the only participant involved talking about his background and views on a number of issues. He was then interviewed four more times when he was at technical college, most recently at age 22. He comes from a Protestant family in a Northern Ireland city and at the first contact he was living with both his parents and older sister. At the time of the first designated interview, aged 18, he was in the middle of doing an advanced GNVQ in business studies at the 'Tech', having passed his ordinary level GNVQ with a distinction. He wanted to work with computers, but preferably in a 'behind the scenes' role, like someone who travels round fixing them. Neville was also very keen on cars and had recently taken and passed his driving test. He said how thrilled he was, and remembered that his mother was very excited for him too. Although they had a close relationship, she was not so pleased when he crashed the family car into a wall!

However, as Neville went on to describe, a couple of weeks after his embarrassing episode with the car, he was in the house with his mother when she collapsed. He tried unsuccessfully to resuscitate her and she died. It was something to do with her heart and totally unexpected because she had been very healthy, never ill, and there were no signs of anything wrong. It was a very traumatic thing to deal with:

> I don't think I ever will [get over it] because the picture that's stuck clear in my head, you know, what happened that day because like I tried CPR and all this you know, and it was just like . . . I can remember as if it was yesterday you know . . . I just have to go on you know, the family just decided to go on you know and not to dwell on the past and to go on. And that was it.

As Neville commented, something like this puts everything else into the shade:

> Everything comes into perspective you know, things that . . . like I crashed our old car on Boxing Day and that just paled in comparison with this you know . . .

Family life was at a standstill as they tried to take in what had happened:

> We were just walking around like zombies you know. We weren't functioning as a team any more. We just wouldn't be bothered you know. It wasn't the fact that we weren't bothered, it was more the fact that we were still grieving type of thing.

Neville's father had taken two weeks off work, during which he read a book on 'bereavement' and decided that they should try and get themselves together by setting up some routine: 'to try get some sort of thing going. Because if you don't like, you'll just fall apart and be finished'. His father also decided that the best thing for them all was to return to work or college. Neville found the first time back at the Tech very hard:

> When I went in the first day and sat through two hours of class and went out to lunch then for about an hour and went up and bought a leather jacket, the one you see sitting on the chair, and came back and said I can't do this. I went home then and came back the next day and then I started back. But it was the first day back after she died that was the hardest. And then after that I kind of was back to full steam then.

He talked of how he was determined to work hard, to keep doing well and get another distinction at college for the sake of his mother. There was also another side to his perseverance, which had emerged in his one-man focus group interview at age 17, when he recounted that when he was about 2 he had been very ill with some kind of virus that had attacked his senses so that he could not move. At the time the doctors had not known what it was and so his parents took him to a healer. Although he recovered, this had left him with some slowness of movement and a problem with coordination, for instance, carrying cups of coffee, or writing well, so he always used a laptop for college work. Reflecting back in the interview, he put his own determination to do well down to his mother:

> My mum had the faith to believe in it, so that's why I try hard . . . Like that there was a miracle really. If my mum hadn't believed I wouldn't be here today . . . I think that if you do try hard enough . . . I think you can make it.

Neville described how his friends turned up trumps when his mother died. They rang up and called round and were generally supportive. He did not always want to be sociable, but he really appreciated their efforts:

> I don't know how many offers I had to go out and everything would be paid for but I just didn't feel like it at that stage you know but it just shows you how good friends are like you know – it was great . . . they helped me through it and they know it too because I told them that many times. And they said it's not because we took pity on you it was because you are a friend.

He had had a girlfriend for a few months and really enjoyed being in what he felt was a steady relationship:

> It was great when I was going steady you know. It was good craic, 'cos you've always got something to look forward to that weekend you know . . . going out there, going to the cinema, bowling alley or something . . . there's always something to do.

But she suddenly cooled off and they split up. He did not know why and felt hurt at the way she did it, but said his mother's death put that into perspective too:

> It was like, och, it's over now you know, and it's not that major like you know, compared to things that have happened to me in the last year so . . .

He and his friends had also planned to go to Spain on holiday in the summer, for which he initially did not have much enthusiasm, but in the event it was just what he needed and they all had a really good time.

Just over a year after his mother's death, aged 19, life had settled down, Neville was doing well in college and his sister was engaged, but he found constant re-minders of his mother, and said that things like photographs 'would trigger me off':

> It's um ... easing up a wee bit. Och, it's hard but you just have to go on and stuff ... I just can't get over it at times ... When it's really hard, it's like losing part of yourself and then you know that part of yourself, and you just have to ... it's like learning to walk again ... I'm finding it a bit harder. Maybe the rest of them are just coping with it or looking as if they're coping with it but I'm not. There's times when I really don't cope at all. You know, I'm in this house nearly every night and maybe I've been working on an assignment and then you know, something just reminds me of my mum or you know, you walk past that hall ...

He and his father had established a good relationship and had developed a way of sharing the housework, which Neville was not always very good at. His father was paying for him to concentrate on his studies and get his education done, and also lent him the car more or less whenever he wanted it. They had an understanding that if he needed money for things like clothes, he just asked his father:

> He says, 'If you need money, just ask me and I'll give it to you', because he doesn't see what me mum sees, or did see. You know, 'You need a new pair of jeans', he wouldn't see that ...

As Neville recounted in the third interview, at age 20, he and his sister Bridget had also had to get used to their father having a new relationship. He had asked them for their permission to 'date' and they had given it:

> We said fine because at the end of the day I could be happy, my sister could be happy, but if he's stuck here on his own like it's not, and she's good for him you know she really is and she's a nice woman too.

But clearly his mother's death still loomed large for Neville and he sometimes drove up to the graveyard car park late at night to talk to her:

> I would just sit in the car – for ten minutes or whatever and just talk and I would come out then a bit refreshed.

There were times when he wished he could get away from everything and start again but he accepted that he liked his course and his family and friends. He was constantly preoccupied with his mother:

> It still hurts like hell and you know, there's nothing you can do. You can't bring her back. You can't change time or anything but it's just a struggle at times and other times, I can cope for a couple of weeks and not really think about her. But you know, the next day I'll be thinking about her non stop just and it goes through my head all of this, you know, what

happened, what – what I did, and what could've have happened, and all this crap and I just can't do anything really about it like ...

Neville achieved a distinction from college – he had heard the news on another summer holiday with his friends and they had all celebrated – then he went on to take a two year HND in business studies and IT. In general he didn't want to go out much, apart from occasionally meeting friends for a drink or to play football or snooker. His sister had recently moved up the road to live with her boyfriend so it was now he and his father at home, but this was no problem, they got on well, and she would often pop in to see them and comment on the state of the housework.

Losing someone so close, and in such a sudden manner, left Neville with underlying concerns for those nearest to him:

> I would be worried about it if he's [father] not up before me in the morning ... or if I shout him and he's not answering me I would be worried about that because I'm worried that, you know, something could happen.

For Neville, the time around the date of losing his mother was always a tough one:

> Well it's eased a bit but at the same time around the eighth of January I'm for nothing, I couldn't go in to do any work in Tech ... in fact when I do get a job I'm going to ask for that day off and just, it's a day that I can't function and it takes me about a week after that to get back to it.

To mark the second anniversary of his mother's death, he had written up the whole event in great detail, which he had shown to his sister but not yet to his father, and had also left it with a tutor at college:

> ... on the eighth of January I sat down at the laptop and wrote the whole thing out, from start to finish ... I just sat down and typed, I can even remember conversations we were having on that day and who came in and if somebody came in and what I said to them and blah, blah. It took me ten pages to write it but it was so, just like somebody lifting a weight off your shoulders because I kept it in for two years and I just thought right, I was meaning to do it but I didn't know when to do it and I thought I'll do it on the anniversary two years on because it means more, do you know what I mean?

Neville was also concerned that his twenty-first birthday, in a few months time, would 'be a sad time' without his mother there to plan a party for him, though he also talked of support from his grannies, uncle and aunt.

Neville spoke in this interview of the ways that he felt he had changed:

> You know, I'm not as outgoing now as I was before but maybe that's just me and I don't drink as much now as I did before. I'm not saying I was an alcoholic before but I would take the car out more often. I think I'm a more emotional person now. You know, something happens on the TV and I'd be in tears like and it wouldn't be that severe but um ... Well, I wouldn't be crying at everything ... but I wouldn't be as strong as I was before. And I find it hard to get motivated most of the time now.

Asked to describe himself now, he said: 'Caring. A caring person who likes cars'. He had clearly changed from the person he was some years previously, who apparently had a fiery temper and was always getting into trouble:

> ... like if somebody came to the door and gave me cheek like you know ... whereas five years ago I would have torn the face off him, f'ing and blinding and all that. I've calmed down now that way ... I still have a bit of a temper but I've just calmed down, I've just grown out of it ...

Questioned on whether there was anything else that was important to him about his identity, he referred to his 'ability to get on with other religions' – his friends at the Tech had come from both Catholic and Protestant backgrounds, but had all got on very well:

> I don't see the sense in us fighting and guns and stuff and killing loyalists and killing Catholics, I don't see the point of it because I have friends living in this estate, I've known them for ten years say and we get on the best and we might have drifted apart because we are at different colleges or different countries or whatever, but we still come back.

His plans were to go on to university after his HND and then get a job in computing, and he would have liked another steady relationship but had so far met no one appropriate. When interviewed nearly two years later, aged 22, Neville had completed his HND course but decided not to pursue university even though he had been offered a place. He felt it was now time he started work, although he was already feeling the disadvantage of never having had any work experience, and felt he had lost some of his previous confidence to do well. His sister had got married, an event that underlined the absence of his mother, whose role on that occasion had been taken by his aunt. He was living at home with his father, with whom he still got on well, but he was anxious that his father might bring his girlfriend to live with them. Neville had let his friends go a bit during the last year or so, and become more isolated and dependent on his family for emotional and practical support. At his most recent contact, he had taken another further education course, his father had married his girlfriend and they had all moved to a house in a different area.

Commentary

It seems that Neville continued with his aims and ambitions, despite not really coming to terms with his mother's death. He did well at college, although his decision not to go to university came as a surprise in the context of his earlier ambitions, and remains something of a puzzle in this analysis, though it perhaps links to his expressed loss of confidence and motivation. While his family and friends have been very important and helped to sustain him through these difficult years, the successive interviews also seemed to suggest that he became more isolated as time went on. He describes himself as having become more emotional and less outgoing, with a loss of confidence and an absence of any steady girlfriend, and he expresses anxiety about his father and sister.

Core themes that recur in the interviews include issues to do with 'coping' (or not) and 'going on' (or not), and the changes he has felt in himself as a result of the death of his mother. The depth of the devastation, and his struggles to deal with this alongside the absence of opportunities to talk, are themes to which he regularly returns in the various interviews. He describes gaps that can't be filled, and the vulnerability he experienced is expressed in terms of having to learn to walk again. Some of these issues are discussed in terms of everyday topics like housework and money, but some are described in directly emotional terms. The death itself, which was clearly a traumatic experience, also continues to preoccupy Neville over the years. While it is hard to find anything positive to say about Neville's accounts in relation to his mother's death, as they change over the years, and while he appears quite an isolated figure in dealing with his emotions, he does recount two strategies that he has developed for himself: namely, visiting the graveyard to talk to his mother, and the major event of writing it all down on the second anniversary of her death. In other ways, though, Neville does describe positive attributes about himself that have developed over time, including a calming down of his fiery temper, and his ability to make friends across the sectarian divides of his community. We are left with the question of whether or not his involvement in the research interviews in itself perhaps provided helpful opportunities for talk that would otherwise not have occurred at all.

Themes from the perspectives of bereaved young people

If we turn now to put these case studies into the context of the whole range of evidence we discussed earlier in this chapter, which may provide qualitative insights into the nature of young people's experiences of bereavement, there are a number of themes that can be distinguished.

The search for meaning

A search for meaning, within young people's accounts of their bereavement experiences, may be understood to refer to broad spiritual or existential issues, such as: beliefs about an afterlife; whether a death had any purpose; whether there is anything to be learned from it at a personal level; and how it may shape a young person's approach to life generally. But the search for meaning might also refer, in a more mundane sense perhaps, to the manner in which people inevitably seek to find a way to be able to think about, or talk about, events in their lives, building on whatever set of assumptions, constructs or expectations individuals already use to build their everyday worlds upon. This latter sense of the search for meaning does not necessarily connote the idea that a death is felt to be meaning*ful* by a young person (although the more existential or spiritual search might seek to find such meaningfulness). But a fundamental characteristic of humans is that people are sense-making enti- ties, so that, with or without a view of death as meaningful, bereavement will inevitably lead to a search for some way to make sense of the event, enabling the individual to incorporate the experience into their ongoing and unfolding 'assumptive world' (Janoff-Bulman 1992), or everyday 'typifications' (Schutz 1954). We will return to this discussion in Chapter 6, but here we can note how, even within the more qualitative evidence that we have considered in this chapter, there is variable scope between different qualitative approaches for perceiving this search for meaning on the part of bereaved individuals. This is, however, one of the strengths of a narrative approach, particularly where narratives have been documented over a period of some time.

In their different ways, each of the young people we have presented as case studies attempt to consider what meaning the bereavement has had for their view of life – in both the more existential sense and the more mundane sense. This is most explicit, probably, with Shirleen and Khattab, although the meanings also shift over the course of their interviews. Their narratives constitute important evidence of the ways in which bereavement experiences may have highly significant implications for a young person's world view without necessarily being experienced as highly disruptive in an emotional or biographical sense.

Brian's views on his life in relation to his father's death also shift at different points, with an emphasis at times on the happy memories of his good relationship with his father, while at other times the sadness is upper- most, leading to the conclusion that his life has been 'unlucky'. In the early interviews with Neville there is a strong appreciation of the discovery that his friends would support him through his bereavement, but by the end of the sequence of interviews, this has dissipated and Neville appears a lonely figure. For Neville, then, the struggle to 'cope' seems to override anything else in terms of how he makes sense of his mother's death.

It is perhaps Maeve's narratives that show the greatest changes over time, from the early shock and threat to her sense of meaning, to the later more general conclusions she has drawn from her experiences. The early interviews after her friends' deaths are thus dominated by a sense of overwhelming emotion felt by Maeve and her peers, which at first they can only deal with by clinging together. But as time goes on, she develops a slightly more reflective view of how these experiences have changed her as a person and shaped her outlook on life generally, to make her 'tougher' in a way that can parallel other life experiences.

What we hope, in addition, is that the case studies can convey, to some degree, the depths and complexities of the different 'realities' that are narrated by these young people regarding their varying experiences of bereavement. Others, writing on other substantive issues, or from other methodological frameworks, have also pointed to the need to understand children and young people's perspectives on their situations, and to see these in the context of longitudinal accounts (Hetherington 2003) (a point to which we return below). In this respect, what these various writers help point towards is the way in which significant events in an individual's personal biography need to be understood by reference to their own pre-existing approach to life, with bereavement a potentially significant – sometimes disruptive – issue for the ways in which young people develop their world views.

Overwhelming feelings

What is more apparent across the range of qualitative materials – autobiographical, psychological, narrative – that we have considered here, is the way in which some bereavements can give rise to an experience of overwhelming emotions (as graphically portrayed in Rebecca's poem on p. viii of this book). And young people may struggle to 'manage' such emotions, let alone make any sense of them. Furthermore, they may feel that their emotions are not acknowledged, and that they have nowhere to express them, or talk about them.

One important feature of the calls made to ChildLine concerns the need children seemed to be expressing to have someone hear them speak of their strong emotions, often very shortly after a death had occurred, and sometimes in very brief calls of one or two minutes (Cross 2002). Other callers often spoke of their surprise and fear at their own feelings, expressing a strong sense of not knowing how to behave. And, while calls that concerned serious suicidal intent were not included in Cross's report (as they were not classified as primarily concerning bereavement), it is noteworthy that nearly 10 per cent spoke of wanting to die.

Furthermore, an issue which pervades much of the work on young people's own perspectives is that of not knowing how to communicate such overwhelming and unknown feelings. Communication can be hampered by a belief that not talking about it is a form of protection – not mentioning things that might upset someone. It is very clear that family members often try to protect one another and maintain collusions of silence. As Neville said in relation to his family relationships, 'Maybe the rest of them are just coping with it, or looking as if they're coping, but I'm not'.

There is also confusion and concern about what constitutes 'normal' grief reactions, and what is 'acceptable' behaviour. Nevertheless, we have to be aware that this theme of communication, while highly suggestive, could lead towards contrasting conclusions: that young people lack opportunities but want to talk (discussed further in Chapter 5), or that it is those young people who value communication who appear in the published evidence available to us. And there is very little evidence that concerns the broad range of young people who have not been particularly identified as bereaved for the purposes of either research studies or interventions. Our case studies offer particularly important evidence about young people generally but, even so, these are individuals who were willing to be repeatedly interviewed, in depth, over several years, as part of a general study of the lives of young people.

Social relationships and social context

A major feature of all the materials we have considered in this chapter is the significance of bereavement in terms of its implications for social relationships and vice versa. In this respect the qualitative evidence crucially focuses our attention on the way in which bereavement experiences occur within a web of pre-existing and ongoing social contexts, which are also quite central to individuals' own perspectives on such life events.

Alongside issues of communication, isolation and loneliness are common themes. Besides the loss of the parent who has died, many young people face secondary losses, such as a breakdown in other relationships (plus loss of innocence, and perhaps loss of role) during the bereavement process (Pennells and Smith 1995). This can be due, in the case of parental death, to the surviving parent being unable to support their children because of their own grief. Young people may also lose friends because their peers do not know how to handle the situation (discussed further in Chapter 5).

But social context is also crucial in a more general sense: of providing clues about how to experience, understand, or manage bereavement, and it is those closest to young people who are likely to be most significant in this regard (Elliott 1999). Wilby (1995), for example, draws on two case studies to highlight different experiences/outcomes occurring within contrasting family cultures. In a broader context again, McNally (2005) explores the way in which the ongoing history of the Troubles in Northern Ireland has framed the understandings of adults bereaved, as a result of the Troubles, of a parent during childhood. But generally, there is very little research which places young people's bereavement experiences into their specific social contexts.

Risk and vulnerability

Both Brian and Neville appear to be vulnerable as they recount their current lives and social contexts, Neville in terms of emotional isolation and Brian in terms of the fact that his bereavement compounded his dependence on his mother, who was herself made more vulnerable. We have no way of knowing whether Neville would have been defined as being 'at risk' by reference to more psychologically or clinically based measures, but we ponder whether anyone around him was aware of the (increasing) depth of his continuing isolation and unhappiness several years on from his mother's death. We are left wondering whether the production of his spontaneous written statement of the trauma of his mother's death helped to remedy this situation.

A further feature of social contexts is that they may put a bereaved young person into direct risk of major harm as a result of bereavement. A particularly disturbing feature of the calls to ChildLine (5 per cent altogether) was the presence of associated problems of abuse and neglect (and, in turn, calls that were primarily categorized as being about physical or sexual abuse mentioned bereavement as a feature of the child's situation): 'Dad came to my bed this morning. He said it wouldn't hurt. Mum died and I miss her' (Cross 2002: 11). The use of alcohol by adults dealing with their own difficult emotions is a regular feature of these calls: 'Mum beats my little brother. She won't listen to me. She didn't drink until my stepdad died'.

At the same time, young people's accounts also point to wider risks of social isolation, bullying and stigma outside family relationships. In a case such as Brian, an underlying vulnerability may be increased by bereavement, while Neville's story highlights how vulnerability may deepen over time.

The significance of time

One clear link that the case studies have with a theme that is raised, but not centralized, in existing published work, is the importance of ongoing issues over time, including as other losses occur in people's lives, which links also with the theme of re-emergence of grief that we identified earlier. One study (Normand *et al.* 1996 cited by Gillies and Neimeyer 2006) has explored the ways in which children and young people's relationship with their deceased parent may change over time in ways that young people themselves may value. In the more quantitative and medicalized empirical work, the implications of bereavement in the longer term are only addressed with regard to studies that seek to establish whether or not the death of a parent during childhood is a risk factor for depression in adult life (see Chapter 4).

How grief is experienced over time within the life course is something we appear to know little about, despite the well-worn reliance on the idea that 'time is a healer'. Morin and Welsh (1996), in their study of adolescent perceptions of death and bereavement in America, found that the most helpful coping strategy was the reminder that time would help, while the least helpful was platitudes such as 'you'll get over it'. The Cruse interactive website for teenagers (discussed in Chapter 5) has a 'timeline' which children can access and add to, about their feelings and experiences at different time points (e.g. on the day of death, one week/month/year later etc.). The variability of experience can be exemplified by one contributor to the timeline who wrote, four years on from the death of her father, followed later by the deaths of her uncle and her cousin: 'the person that said time is a healer I'd like to meet and probally shoot because they obviously knew nothing!'. Similar reactions are also apparent in the analysis of calls to ChildLine (Cross 2002).

Retrospective accounts of bereavement in childhood/teenage years show how grief may re-emerge over time at significant points in later life (Pennells and Smith 1995; Elliott 1999, and see also the Cruse 'timeline' web page at www.rd4u.org.uk). Time is also a significant issue in the ChildLine calls in the opposite direction, with regard to the immediacy of the shock and bewilderment expressed by some of these young callers, one third of whom called within two weeks of the death, and some from the hospital immediately after the death.

Interventions

Only one of our five case studies had experienced any particular intervention or opportunities for discussion of their bereavement provided to them by any formal service providers, although we can also see their own efforts to 'cope'. This points to the need for opportunities to talk among existing informal social relationships, but the difficulties in social relationships, and lack of opportunities to talk, are major themes to arise from this exploration of the 'voices' of young people (as we have discussed above). This raises issues about social attitudes generally towards bereavement, and the possibilities of educating young people in this area, both in relation to highly disruptive bereavements (such as Neville's), and other experiences of bereavement (such as Shirleen's and Khattab's). As we saw in Chapter 1, and as we have tried to demonstrate through our selection of case studies, bereavement experiences may constitute a highly significant feature of the life course of the majority of young people. Furthermore, such concerns about social isolation and opportunities for interventions also point to the importance of referral processes being available to young people, with or without their parents acting as gatekeepers to services and support (issues to which we return in Chapter 5).

Young people's lack of power

While Cross (2002) describes the calls to ChildLine in terms of the difficulties bereaved young people may have in understanding what they are feeling, she also suggests that the feelings expressed are no different in kind to the sorts of feelings experienced by adults in similar circumstances. Instead, she suggests, the differences centre more on the lack of power experienced by young people combined, frequently, with a sense of exclusion from decisions being made (and see also some of the case studies in McNally 2005). This points to a key feature of the way in which young people's experiences of bereavement may raise particular issues as a result of their specific social positioning – both among their immediate social relationships, and within the context of wider institutional structures.

Conclusions

While much of the qualitative evidence we have available to us concerning young people's experiences of bereavement focuses on the deaths of particularly significant family members (most notably the death of a parent), the case studies we have presented here draw our attention to the range of ways in which bereavement may constitute a highly significant feature of young people's life experiences. This is so, firstly, with regard to the categories of relationships involved. Thus, the case studies include young people for whom the loss of friends and more distant relatives, as well as parents, constituted major features of their life narratives. This is in line with the more quantitative evidence presented in Chapter 1, which points to the statistical as well as the emotional significance of a wide range of bereavements in the lives of young people, including friends, wider family relationships, partners, children and pets. In the calls to ChildLine (Cross 2002), the categories of loss primarily centred on parents and grandparents, with death of a mother being the single most frequently cited category. But other forms of loss also included siblings, friends (including partners and ex-partners), pets (particularly among younger children), miscarriages and abortions.

But, besides the range of losses, these qualitative materials also draw our attention to the range of possible reactions among bereaved young people. Thus one particularly significant insight concerns the striking evidence of how apparently similar bereavements may shift individual experiences in quite opposite directions – something that may be lost within more quantitative studies of 'outcomes'.

In the following chapters, we turn to consider these quantitative studies in their own right. In doing so, we may find that some themes, and categories of loss, that are highlighted by the more qualitative evidence, are lost from view. Nevertheless, some of the themes discussed above are receiving increasing attention from the more structured research studies, even if this is a fairly recent development, particularly as the more quantitative approaches seek to explore in greater complexity why individuals differ with regard to some of the 'outcomes' of bereavement. This is the case with regard to issues of familial and cultural context, and also with the issue of secondary and multiple losses.

In other respects, however, there may be some striking convergence between the evidence of the quantitative and qualitative studies. In some ways, the case studies we present here can be used, as others before them, to illustrate themes in the quantitative literature, whether it is the gender dynamics of Neville's emotional distance from his father, and both his and Brian's loss of steady relationships with girlfriends in the years following the deaths of their parents, or whether it is the striking way they both talk about wanting to do well educationally to please their dead parent, while Neville then drops out of higher education despite his success in his qualifications. In these respects, the qualitative material can serve to deepen our understanding of the lived experiences that may underlie some of the statistical patterns. It is the statistical patterns that we turn to next.

4 Bereavement as a 'risk' factor in young people's lives

Introduction

In earlier chapters we have been concerned to consider the theoretical and cultural frameworks (potentially) underpinning the conjunction of 'bereavement' and 'young people', and the qualitative evidence available concerning how young people themselves 'voice' their experiences of bereavement. In this chapter, we turn to the more quantitative evidence to ask the question of whether bereavement has been identified as a 'risk' factor in the lives of young people, in terms not of the nature of experiences as voiced by young people themselves, but of bereavement as an 'objective' variable that has been investigated to see if it has deleterious implications for the lives of young people, as identified and operationalized by researchers.

In contemporary western societies 'risk' is often viewed as something predictable and calculable. As a result, an emphasis on risk assessment and evaluation is commonplace. However, the concept of 'risk' – and people's own perceptions of risk – are complex. Moreover, in a 'risk society' the uncertainties associated with risk are recognized (see Beck 1992; Marris 1996; Giddens 1999), even alongside the continuing belief in, and search for, knowledge that will enable us to extend the control that may be possible through scientific understanding. This points to the social construction of the concept of 'risk' underlying the research studies. From a medical orientation, risk research is concerned with 'the identification of factors that accentuate or inhibit disease and deficiency states, and the processes that underlie them' (Garmezy 1994: 9). In the current UK policy context, risk is particularly discussed in terms of factors that increase vulnerability to, or promote protection against, features of social exclusion (Bynner 2001). And alongside such issues of 'risk', recent years have seen an increase in interest in issues of 'resilience', understood as 'a dynamic process of encompassing positive adaptation within the context of significant adversity' (Luthar *et al.* 2000: 543). (We return to issues of resilience later in the chapter.) Additionally, throughout this discussion, we also need to be aware that 'risk' research assumes that some outcomes can be classed as 'beneficent' and others as 'negative', but are the implications of bereavement more equivocal than this allows for? As Small and Memmo point out, 'social, cultural and historical forces play a large role in any evaluation of outcomes as positive or negative' (2004: 4). And, as Craib discusses, some of the most significant implications of bereavement may not be open to scrutiny in this way at all: 'I am not sure how the beginnings of an understanding of suffering, which is itself a suffering, could be measured in an outcome study' (1994: 32).

As discussed in Chapter 2, death, dying and bereavement may be seen as particularly difficult issues in the context of the modern project of progress through rational thought and control of our own destinies. And 'youth' as a social category itself implicates particular ideas about 'risk' and self-control, with institutional processes for monitoring whether certain individual young people may be 'at risk' of various outcomes or events that are considered undesirable: 'The concept of "at risk" depends on the idea that a majority of young people are "on target", making the transitions towards adulthood in the appropriate way' (Wyn and White 1997: 22).

The nature of the evidence

Alongside such broad theoretical issues concerning the meaning of 'risk', there are important methodological and theoretical variations in the studies we will review in this chapter. Some research, more oriented to social policy, is interested in the teenage years as an important time for 'transition' (as discussed in Chapter 2), and so considers bereavement in relation to measured aspects of 'successful' transition experiences, such as age of leaving school or home, educational qualifications and employment status. In this regard, the teenage years may be the time at which childhood 'outcomes' start to be measured, as young people approach their adult lives.

Those studies that are concerned with the teenage years as an important life phase in their own right tend to be based in the more psychological or medical literature and to focus on outcomes that are concerned with health and well-being, such as depression, self-esteem and suicidal tendencies. For example, one well-regarded study of this type is that of Silverman and Worden (Worden 1996), who looked specifically at parentally bereaved children where the parents had been living together prior to the death. This study, based in a particular (largely Roman Catholic) location in Boston, USA, identified appropriate families through funeral directors, and was able to contact almost all relevant families. However, only 51 per cent agreed to participate, and Worden aptly observes that 'We must assume that there may be some bias in favour of people who see value in talking about their grief' (p. 4).

As well as following up these children up to two years after the death of their parent, the research also involved 70 control children matched on key characteristics with the bereaved families. At the time of their bereavement, 52 per cent of the children in the study were adolescents, and this proportion of course increased over the period of the research. As a research design, then, this study has some important strengths, but not many of the psychologically or medically oriented studies are able to show this sort of rigour, often relying on even more restricted samples, or lacking in control group comparisons.

In asking the question, 'does bereavement constitute a risk factor for undesirable outcomes in young people's lives?' there are three main methodological approaches that can be taken to researching this issue with respect to the sample population:

1   To consider information about large numbers of young people who have been randomly selected from the population of young people generally, and to investigate whether there is a statistically significant association between undesirable outcomes and the occurrence of bereavement, and whether there are grounds for inferring that such an association represents a causal relationship. These studies have generally been undertaken primarily by sociologists, and the aim may be to provide baseline knowledge by which to profile children and young people in the general population likely to experience particular life events, and whether these involve increased probability, or 'risk', of particular outcomes. Such findings may then have policy relevance. As we shall discuss later, these studies have rarely focused on bereavement *per se*, although many contain analyses relevant to bereavement issues.

2   To identify young people or adults who are known to have been bereaved, and consider the incidence of problematic events in their lives (either prospectively or retrospectively), ideally with a control group for comparison, or by comparison with what would be expected by reference to what is known about the relevant population generally. This approach can incorporate both clinical case studies of very small numbers of bereaved individuals, and community-based samples of rather larger numbers of bereaved individuals, identified through a variety of means (such as Worden's study, 1996). These studies are generally oriented towards intervention and mitigation of undesirable outcomes, framed within a largely medical perspective.

3   To consider young people who have been identified as having manifested problematic outcomes in their lives, and look back to see if there is a higher incidence of prior bereavement than would be expected from what is known about young people generally. Such studies are most likely to be found in the social policy or social work literature, although they may also be based in a more therapeutic/medical model.

The great majority of the studies, that we accessed through the systematic bibliographic searches that we undertook, fall into the second approach, where samples of individuals known to have been bereaved were investigated, identified either through clinical populations, or through surveys of community populations. There is also a major body of work that takes the first approach, analysing the possibilities of different outcomes in the lives of large-scale samples of young people generally, who have been followed up over many years. There are also some, more isolated, studies that fall into the third category.

As with any form of social research, all of these approaches are subject to a variety of methodological critiques and weaknesses. For example, in relation to the large-scale longitudinal data sets (category 1 above), questions have been raised about the adequacy of the data sets and samples involved. Studies focused on individuals known to have been bereaved (category 2 above) have also been critiqued with regard to the nature of the samples, while the last approach (category 3 above) may be hampered by our lack of knowledge of the prevalence rates of different forms of bereavement in the population of young people generally (see Chapter 1). We return to such specific methodological issues later in this chapter.

There are also complex issues at stake about the meanings of 'causality' in these varied methodologies. In the large-scale studies, 'outcome' may arguably be quite a misleading term to use, unless the reader has a good understanding of the statistically based reasoning behind the models being tested in the data. As Sweeting *et al.* point out in a footnote: 'The term "outcome" here is used as a shorthand for dependent variables in a statistical sense, and is not meant to imply that we assume direction of causality *from* family life *to* any of these variables' (1998: 42). Such caveats may, however, be lost on a non-specialist audience. As Harrison and Harrington (2001) discuss, any associations found between bereavement and a particular outcome (in their study, depression) cannot simply be assumed to reflect a causal relationship, and might, indeed, sometimes be appropriately described as merely 'statistical markers' (Bynner 2001: 286). Hence, it may be a complex matter to establish the processes underlying any such statistical associations.

Rutter (2000) provides an extended discussion of this issue in relation to psychosocial influences generally for development, including the various tensions between environmental and genetic influences, and interactive causality between different processes over time. For example, while experience of major disasters may have 'a substantial effect on emotional psychopathology' (p. 388), it is also apparent that such psychopathology may increase the probability of being exposed to these types of disasters. In relation to children and young people, particularly, there may be a tendency to assume that the child or young person is subject to causal factors that impinge upon them 'externally', rather than viewing the individual child as an active participant in their social relationships, such that the causal process may be reversed, or at least seen as interactive. For example, studies vary as to whether they give any consideration to the possibility that parenting style may *reflect* the child's characteristics as much as it *shapes* them.

A further major issue concerns the point in time at which an 'outcome' can be said to have occurred, and to be measured. Indeed, some writers have suggested that 'if there is literally *no* predictability in the course of bereavement from one day to the next, then the entire premise of measuring it might be called into question' (Neimeyer and Hogan 2001: 111). In a rather different context from that of bereavement, Erlenmeyer-Kimling *et al.* (1990: 362), in a longitudinal investigation of risk factors for schizophrenia, found that outcome measures could vary a good deal according to when the 'outcome' was measured, pointing to 'the dilemma ... of defining what constitutes "outcome" and when outcome occurs'. Consequently, different individual children could be assessed to be at risk in quite variable ways over time. The possibility has been raised, for example, of 'sleeper effects', such that the individual child might show low levels of short-term outcomes, but might develop other reactions after a period of time (as in relation to divorce, see Hetherington 2003). A major finding of Worden and Silverman's study (Worden 1996) was that children might experience more signs of negative consequences at two years than they did at four months or one year.

Some researchers have used retrospective designs to investigate outcomes (e.g. Tremblay and Israel 1998; Worden *et al.* 1999). Robins and Rutter (1990) argue that retrospective studies can be used if the topics of investigation have been tested for reliability, but also point out that some issues will systematically shape characteristics of those who continue to participate in the research. Studies also vary considerably in the extent to which they incorporate or depend upon any subjective evaluations of the significance of a particular bereavement. Davies (1991), for example, discusses the extent to which children and adults report behaviours that they themselves retrospectively attribute to the loss of a sibling in childhood, such that they at least impute causal significance to their bereavement experiences.

In terms of the categories of 'outcomes' being considered, it is also clear across the various literatures that it is generally outcomes that are regarded as undesirable that are the focus of attention (Rodgers and Pryor 1998), particularly in the general longitudinal studies. In the context of research on divorce, Amato comments in this regard, 'If more studies explicitly searched for positive outcomes, then the number of studies documenting beneficial effects of divorce would almost certainly be larger' (2000: 1274).

In examining these studies, then, we have to bear in mind that any specific research study must be regarded as incorporating the strengths and weaknesses of the particular methodology on which it is based, since all choices about research methods entail gains and losses of varying kinds. Overall, much of the evidence is confusing and contradictory. Furthermore, the complexity of the data is demonstrated by the ways in which individual researchers are not always consistent or clear within their treatment or discussion of their own data. In considering some of the details of these inconsistencies, we may perhaps learn more about how to clarify such issues for future research and discussion, pointing to the need for more complex understandings.

In the following two sections of this chapter, we consider studies that treat 'bereavement' as a single variable, in isolation, and consider whether such an experience *per se* increases the probability of certain outcomes in the lives of young people, and into adulthood. In the next section, we consider such outcomes in terms of mental health and more positive psychological measures; the main literature here is based in medical and psychiatric research of samples of bereaved young people (the second methodological approach outlined above), which has considered bereavement as a possible factor in the aetiology of subsequent health problems, and thus identifiable as a threat to well-being. We then turn to examine evidence concerning a range of social outcomes in the lives of young people. Here we rely mainly on the first methodological approach outlined above, largely (but not exclusively) by reference to UK longitudinal and cohort studies of children through the teenage years into adulthood,[1] some of which have considered bereavement experiences. While a direct focus on bereavement issues in this literature is rare, there is, by contrast, an extensive and sophisticated literature that considers the loss of a parent through divorce/separation, with regard to a variety of outcomes. These longitudinal studies will be the primary focus of the second section beginning on p. 00, along with some further studies based on populations of problematic young people (the third methodological approach outlined above). We will then return to a consideration of some of the methodological difficulties found in these particular studies, before turning to the complexity of cross-cutting and contextual issues that may help shape or mediate any outcomes, which may underlie some of the complexities of the research findings, and which may help build towards more sophisticated models and understandings. Finally we offer a concluding discussion in the light of the evidence available, and consider how research in this area might go forward.

---

[1] Further details of these studies can be found at www.cls.ioe.ac.uk/Cohort/mainncds.htm.

Bereavement as a risk factor in relation to medical and psychological outcomes

Medical studies of, young people and bereavement have tended to focus on the clinical assessment of 'the bereaved adolescent' as an individual, or the epidemiological assessment of bereavement in adolescence as a public health issue. Quite different methodologies are associated with each of these approaches to bereavement as a medical issue, the findings of which may or may not be seen as complementary. Indeed, at times the debates have led to some impassioned controversies. Here we concentrate on pathological/ normal outcomes of bereavement, and aspects of well-being and mental health.

As we shall see later in relation to disruptive or criminal behaviours, mental health problems may sometimes be discussed as an alternative outlet from 'acting out' behaviours, as a result of family disruption. Gersten *et al.* (1991: 496) also suggest there are quite different mental health patterns associated with different forms of family disruption, such that 'The different relationships of parental death and divorce with depression and conduct disorder strongly suggest distinct risk situations that cannot be combined under a common concept of loss' (p. 496). They thus point to the possibility that these different types of parental loss are associated with different sorts of problematic outcome that may be in some senses seen as 'alternative' outlets for the expression of loss. Nevertheless, many studies treat all forms of parental 'loss' together. Furthermore, in more general populations, there is evidence that 'internalizing' and 'externalizing' mental health symptoms may often occur together, particularly if they started to manifest themselves in adolescence (Fleming and Offord 1990 cited by Seiffge-Krenke 2000), possibly as a result of overlapping risk factors: 'Different types of stressors as well as the general stress level of cumulative changes may affect the adolescent and lead to a generalized and varied picture of coexistent disorders' (Seiffge-Krenke 2000: 677 citing Caron and Rutter 1991).

In considering the empirical research literature on bereavement as a 'risk' factor for the physical or mental health of adolescents, we find a particular focus on selected aspects of health and well-being, such as enuresis (e.g. Douglas 1973; Maclean and Kuh 1991; Wadsworth 1991), while other possible outcomes, such as anxiety levels, are neglected. Some of the medical literature is primarily concerned with the implications of bereavement over quite a short time period (unlike the longitudinal research studies considered later, below). The two main areas we consider here are risks for depression and the implications for self-concept.

Depression and general mental health risks

Depression has been a primary focus for research into childhood bereavement and, as discussed above, may sometimes be theorized as resulting from the internalization of grief reactions, rather than the more externalizing reaction of aggressive, disruptive or delinquent behaviours. Depression also needs to be recognized as theoretically distinct from complicated grief (Prigerson 2005), although this is not often discussed in the literature. Indeed, some writers suggest that:

> It is possible that the manifestations of problematic adjustment to the loss of a parent are more subtle than those assessed by [standardized measures of anxiety and depression]. Incorporating other measures, such as a clinical diagnostic assessment, might more comprehensively identify children who experienced difficulty adjusting to parental death.
>
> (Christ 2000: 17)

A further key issue is whether or not research is primarily concerned with depression that is measured as clinically pathological, or with lower levels of experienced depression or psychological distress. In the context of divorce research, Kelly has argued that researchers have been inclined to confuse children's expressions of pain with indices of pathology, and that pain is a 'normal' feature of life: '[children] reported considerable distress in reflecting upon their parents' divorce. However, painful reflections on a difficult past are not the same as an inability to feel and function competently in the present' (2003: 249).[2]

The likelihood of bereavement leading to increased risk of depression is an issue about which there is a marked division and uncertainty in the literature, although the debate is often framed more widely in terms of the long-term risk of clinical depression in adult life associated with the experience of parental bereavement during childhood. We will consider this literature here alongside the more specific research on adolescent experiences, since it relates to the issue of problems that may impinge on adolescent mental health, as part of the overall life course.

There are thus differing understandings concerning what weight to place on any findings of depression, whether depression (objectively measured or otherwise) is understood as problematic or not, and requiring intervention or

---

[2] And see Gillies and Neimeyer (2006) for a recent general discussion of how pain and 'distress', as a result of bereavement, may relate to other outcomes such as 'personal growth' in complex ways.

not. In terms of the *prevalence* of distress and/or depressive symptoms in the short to medium term following a significant bereavement, Harrington and Harrison suggest that 'sadness, crying and withdrawal occur in less than 50% of cases' (1999: 230). While these findings might indicate that we should be careful not to expect that all bereaved adolescents will necessarily experience deep grief and emotional reactions to bereavement, this would not seem to indicate an insubstantial issue for a considerable minority. In a review of relevant literature concerning *parentally bereaved* children, Dowdney seems to make a different emphasis when she suggests that 'Interviews with bereaved children and adolescents reveal marked affective responses to parental death including crying, sadness, anger, guilt and despair' (2000: 821).

In a much cited early study that sought to establish children's responses to parental bereavement, using a community-based sample of 2–17-year-olds, 13 months after the death of their parent, Van Eerdewegh *et al.* (1982) found higher levels of dysphoria and minor depression than among controls, but not severe forms of depression. In a later community based study of 8–15-year-olds in one part of the USA, Gersten *et al.* (1991) identified those who had experienced parental death during the previous two years, where the parent was aged between 25 and 50 and was survived by a spouse. They found clear evidence of an increased risk of depression, 7.5 times higher than in the control group. This finding held true irrespective of the gender of the parent or child, and irrespective of whether the child was under or over 11 at time of death. However, the rate of major depression was twice as high for 12–16-year-olds as for 8–12-year-olds, and was twice as prevalent among girls than boys. These authors also argue that depression is much more commonly a risk for bereaved children than for children whose parents have divorced, suggesting that conduct disorder is more commonly found among divorced children, where the associated gender effect is reversed.

Other writers (e.g. Black 1993; Servaty and Hayslip 2001) have similarly pointed to increased levels of depression among bereaved adolescents. In Silverman and Worden's study of parentally bereaved children and young people over a period of two years (Worden 1996, discussed earlier), the four most common emotional expressions were sadness, anxiety, guilt and anger. By the second anniversary, two thirds of the children and young people said they still cried occasionally, and at this point in time, bereaved adolescents showed more anxiety, depression and worry about their families than their matched controls. Overall, Worden reports that 65 per cent of the children and young people in their study were never assessed as being 'at risk' over the two-year period of the research. On the other hand, one third of the bereaved children in this study were 'found to be at some degree of risk for high levels of emotional and behavioural problems' (1996: 16).

Not all studies find evidence of raised levels of clinical depression, however, and, as noted above, authors may thus vary considerably in the interpretations they put on the evidence (see e.g. Lutzke *et al.* 1997; Sandler *et al.* 1997; Tremblay and Israel 1998, in relation to parentally bereaved children). Some differences in the findings of different studies may relate to variations in the samples studied. For example, among a community-based sample of 9–17-year-olds drawn predominantly from minority ethnic groups, Thompson *et al.* (1998) found that almost a quarter of the bereaved scored in the clinical distress range. Whereas a study of children bereaved of a parent through cancer, drawn from largely white, middle-class, two-parent households (Christ 2000), found that 1 in 15 children showed either a 'compromised' or 'symptomatic' grieving response, with 14–17 per cent falling outside the range of 'normal outcomes'.

In the UK, using a different methodology, some general cohort studies have also found parental bereavement to constitute a risk factor for the psychological well-being of teenagers. The analysis by Ely et al (2000) of two different cohorts (in Scotland using the same cohort as that studies by Sweeting et al 1998, and in Britain using the 1970 BSC data) thus found an association between family structure and risk to psychological well-being, with parental death constituting a greater risk factor than parental separation in this regard.

Dowdney concludes, in her general review of this literature: 'The extent to which depression will be higher amongst bereaved children than in a demographically matched control group remains unknown' (2000: 821) and that:

> ... children do experience grief, sadness and despair following parental death. Mild depression is frequent. However, *when clinically referred children are excluded*, psychiatric disorder characterises only a very small minority of children ... Most commonly, bereaved children present with a wide range of emotional and behavioural symptoms that constitute a nonspecific disturbance. One in five is likely to manifest such disturbance at a level sufficient to justify referral to specialist services ... Inconsistencies in the literature relate to rates of disorder or disturbance rather than to the manner in which children manifest distress.
>
> (2000: 827–9, emphasis added)

Dowdney also suggests that depression following bereavement may show specific features different from other forms of depression.

In reviewing evidence concerning *sibling bereaved* adolescents, both Hogan and DeSantis (1994), and Davies (1998) conclude that several studies point to sibling bereavement as a strong indicator of psychological problems. Worden *et al.* (1999) suggest that around 25 per cent of sibling as well as parentally bereaved children may be considered to be at risk in the first year after bereavement. Again, however, findings are not always consistent and estimates of the numbers of bereaved siblings affected can range from 9 to 87 per cent (Davies 1998). Furthermore, Davies suggests, it is sometimes difficult to distinguish between 'normal grieving' reactions and maladjustment as such.

Studies of *bereavement of a peer* are still largely undeveloped, and tend to rely quite haphazardly on opportunistic or volunteer samples, often of American college students (e.g. O'Brien *et al.* 1991; Schachter 1992; Ringler and Hayden 2000). The vast majority of peer bereavements in these studies have concerned traumatic or violent deaths – as with our case study of Maeve in Chapter 3. As we saw with Maeve, reactions to such deaths may go deep and last for many years, including depression (Schneiderman 1993) and suicidal thoughts, or drug or school problems (Ringler and Hayden 2000). Brent *et al.* (1993) found that depressive reactions among adolescents, after exposure to suicide by a friend or acquaintance, appeared to be bona fide major depression, occurring as a complication of the bereavement. The intensity or duration of associated feelings may not necessarily reflect the closeness of the relationship (O'Brien *et al.* 1991), making this quite a difficult bereavement to assess or research among young people acquainted with a peer who has died.

While Harrington and Harrison argue that parental bereavement does not feature as 'a major risk factor for mental disorder in children' (1999: 230) (discussed above), their own subsequent community-based research data (Harrison and Harrington 2001) clearly point to an association between a *variety of bereavements* and measured depressive symptoms. This study investigated the prevalence of depressive symptoms in adolescents aged 11–16 years at two different schools in the North of England, and found that the loss of a person reported as a close relative or friend was associated with more depressive symptoms. For the deaths of adult relatives, such bereavement was significantly mediated by the implications of the death for (self-reported) subsequent changes in the young person's life, but for deaths of siblings or peers, the strong association with depressive symptoms was not mediated in this way.

Using a different methodological approach, Meltzer *et al.* (2000) carried out a general survey of the mental health of 5–15-year-olds overall in England, Scotland and Wales. Bereavements of differing types were included in the analysis of stressful life events that were associated with various types of mental disorder (namely, conduct disorders, emotional disorders and hypekinetic disorders). Significant associations were found between mental disorder and death of a parent, sibling or close friend, but not with the death of a grandparent or pet.

Besides depression experienced during the early period after bereavement, various writers have considered further questions about how grief may change *over time*. Harrison and Harrington found that 'Deaths that had occurred more than 5 years before were just as likely to be associated with depressive symptoms as deaths that had occurred more recently' (2001: 162).

Worden's study of parentally bereaved children and young people found their 'risk' status (assessed on the basis of scores on an inventory of emotional/behavioural problems) increased between the first and second anniversary of the death:

> This large and significant effect [at two years but not at one year] was one of the most important findings from the study. It suggests that there is a 'late effect' of bereavement for a significant minority of those school-age children, and emphasises the importance of regular follow-up assessments of children over a longer period of time.
>
> (1996: 98)

In a *general* longitudinal study of a community of 5–18-year-olds concerning the risks of major long-term depression, Reinherz *et al.* (1993) found that among depressed girls particularly there were more reports of stressful life events, including the death of a parent. Similarly, when focusing on depression as a feature of the transition to adulthood (at ages 18 and 21), Reinherz *et al.* (1999) again found death of a parent to be a significant risk factor for women, but not for men.

Among sibling bereaved adolescents, some studies (including Guerriero and Fleming 1985 cited by Balk 1995; Balmer 1992 cited by Fleming and Balmer 1996) found that depression decreased over time. By contrast, others (Hogan and Greenfield 1991 cited by Hogan and DeSantis 1994) did not find any lessening of grief among sibling bereaved adolescents with high levels of grief, even 18 months to five years after the death. These authors also discuss the work of Balk (1983) who found that 33–50 per cent of sibling bereaved adolescents had enduring reactions 4–84 months after death, including depression, anger, guilt and confusion. Davies (1998) also suggests that some of the consequences (not all of them negative) of sibling bereavement may increase rather than decline over time, including withdrawal, anxiety and sadness.

Overall, then, with regard to the implications of parental bereavement for distress and depression during the *teenage years as such*, the existing evidence seems to suggest that crying, distress and depressive symptoms are widespread occurrences, concerning perhaps 50–66 per cent of parentally bereaved children and young people, and this is not just a very short-term phenomenon. The evidence also seems to point to a figure of between 20 and 30 per cent of children and young people being regarded as 'at risk' to a degree that might indicate a need for intervention. Among those few studies that have included control group comparisons, these figures are higher than among control groups, and this association is higher than would be expected by chance. Research on sibling bereavement is suggestive of similar levels, but evidence of distress/depression in relation to other categories of bereavement is too limited to draw conclusions, although there is certainly suggestive evidence that bereavement of a peer may also be associated with depression.

Awareness of the possibility of such ongoing and longer-term implications of bereavement may be particularly important in the lives of young people, since earlier bereavements in their lives may either be unknown to those around them currently, or the significance of such losses may be expected to have subsided. As we saw with Neville in Chapter 3, this may be far from the reality.

In the broader literature about the *long-term* implications of childhood parental bereavement for *adult* mental health, the putative link with depression has a substantial history, dating back to the 1960s (Dowdney 2000), including work by Black (1978, 1993), Birtchnell (1972) and Agid *et al.* (1999). In a more recent study, Mack (2001) used large-scale general data sets available from the American National Survey of Families and Households to investigate high levels of depression among adults. The results pointed to raised levels of depression among adults who had experienced parental death during childhood, in comparison with *both* those brought up in intact families and those who had experienced parental divorce during childhood.

However, studies of the more general populations in the UK longitudinal data sets (primarily the National Child Development Study and the Medical Research Council's 1946 Cohort Study, discussed further below) do not necessarily report consistent evidence of such long-term effects, in terms of direct correlations between childhood bereavement and adult depression. Maclean and Wadsworth (1988), for example, found no association between parental death in childhood and measures of emotional well-being at age 36. However, elsewhere Wadsworth (1991) reports that the measure of emotional state used for adults at age 36 was indeed associated with parental death among those with the highest scores. More recently, Schoon and Montgomery (1997), using more sophisticated statistical modelling to analyse these data sets, concluded that death of a parent in childhood (before age 7) was not associated with an increased risk of adult depression. In the USA, a study by Kessler *et al.* (1997), based on the National Comorbidity Survey, also did not find a long-term association between parental bereavement and major depression in adulthood, but did find a relationship with mood disorders.

The complexities of these various contradictory findings concerning the risk of childhood bereavement for long-term depression and wider mental health problems in adulthood, and the possible explanations for them (both theoretical and methodological), defy any straightforward conclusions: 'There are still many questions regarding why it is that some individuals are resilient while others are vulnerable and go on to develop long-term problems' (Worden 1996: 105). A link with depression, both in the teenage years and more long-term, is certainly found in many studies, but there are some notable exceptions to this picture (Lutzke *et al.* 1997).

Protagonists from both sides of the debate concur to some extent, however, in pointing to the likely – or possible – relevance of other mediating factors. Thus Black (1993: 2) suggests that 'other causes for the association between adult depression and childhood bereavement cannot be ruled out', while Harrington and Harrison (1999: 230) write: 'If a link does exist between early parental death and adult depression, then it is probably due to the association between parental death and other risk factors such as lack of adequate parenting'.

We will return to such complexities later in this chapter, but next we consider some of the possible implications of bereavement for other features of the emotional experiences of young people, both negatively and positively experienced.

Self-concept and more 'positive' outcomes

Not all outcomes from bereavement experiences are necessarily regarded as unequivocally negative (Frantz *et al.* 2001). There may, for example, be scope for individuals to gain a different – perhaps more realistic – perspective on life, or a sense of increased strength or maturity in the face of adversity, to develop more spiritual beliefs or a deeper appreciation of the value of their significant relationships – as when Shirleen (Chapter 3) took care to spend time with her grandparents after the death of her great grandfather. More prosaically, individuals may benefit from the ending of a conflictual or abusive relationship. General research on risk and resilience in the lives of young people has raised the possibility of a 'steeling effect' occurring, by which earlier adversity may lead to greater resilience in dealing with later hardships (Small and Memmo 2004). Some researchers have thus paid particular attention to the implications of bereavement for enhanced self-concept and self-esteem among young people. The issues here are again complex, however, pointing to ambivalences and interactive effects.

Fleming and Balmer (1996) suggest that the evidence points to an absence of decline, and maybe an increase in feelings of self-worth and sense of personal maturity after the death of a sibling or other family member. Balk (1995) in particular has paid this issue considerable attention in relation to sibling bereavement in adolescence. In his own work, he found that such young people either came close, or had better, scores on psychological scales measuring positive self-concept, when compared with 'normal' adolescents, and also higher value scores on morality scales (Balk 1983). However, he also found great variation with regard to this issue, alongside reports of continued confusion, suicidal thoughts, fearfulness and eating difficulties among some individuals.

Martinson *et al.* (1987), in another study of sibling bereavement, found higher self-concept scores than among the control group, even seven to nine years after the death (discussed by Hogan and DeSantis 1994), although in a later publication Martinson and Campos (1991) suggest that the long-term effects of sibling bereavement could be very variable. But Birenbaum *et al.*

(1989–90), by contrast, found almost no indication of positive outcomes in their study of sibling bereaved children, either on adaptive functioning or social competency scales, up to one year after the death. Balk also considers the possibility of *inter*active effects between self-concept and adjustment to bereavement, citing the work of Hogan and Greenfield as showing that 'enduring grief symptoms are associated with poor self-concept' (Balk 1995: 176). Balk posits that a high self-concept may enable people to cope with grief better over time (as regards intensity of reported grief), and vice versa.

Worden's work on parentally bereaved children and young people found mixed outcomes in terms of self-perceptions. At one year after the death, three quarters of the children and young people said they felt more 'grown up' as a result of the bereavement experience, and this was especially true of boys and adolescents. How to evaluate this is not entirely clear, however, since adolescent boys were especially likely to report that they were told to act more grown up after their parent's death. Elsewhere, Worden suggests that 'Bereaved children believed they were less able to effect change than their non-bereaved counterparts ... [and] it is difficult to avoid the supposition that this difference had something to do with the death of their parent' (1996: 70). This finding was particularly the case with children whose mother had died, or whose surviving parent was depressed and/or in poor health, or whose families had experienced several losses or changes during the year after the death. This did not improve over time, and by two years 'there was a large and significant difference between the self-esteem scores of the bereaved and the non-bereaved, with bereaved children reporting significantly lower self-worth' (1996: 71).

Tyson-Rawson (1996), also discussing parentally bereaved adolescents, draws on the work of Carse and Silverman to suggest that bereavement may lead to earlier maturity and 'can become a powerful motive for resolving the developmental tasks of adolescence' (1996: 159). Nevertheless, her own work (on paternally bereaved adolescents) suggests they may also feel more vulnerable and less in control.

This (fairly limited) literature on self-esteem, self-concept and bereavement overall seems to point to some differences between the experiences of parentally and sibling bereaved young people. Given the discussion by Worden about the significance of additional factors such as several life changes, it may be that some parental deaths in particular have a major impact on young people's life experiences, in ways that may not be found to be so widespread in relation to sibling deaths,[3] and which then undermine the individual's self-concept and sense of control.

---

[3] Although it is apparent that sibling deaths can also carry financial implications for households – see Corden *et al.* (2001).

Bereavement as a 'risk' factor for social adjustment in youth transitions

One of the comments sometimes made about children who have been bereaved is that they have had to 'grow up too fast', implying that their childhood has been curtailed. The concept of 'pseudomaturity' may be relevant in this context (Newcomb 1996 cited by Rodgers and Pryor 1998) in relation to possible evidence of children from bereaved families moving through transitions at earlier ages than their peers. While there may be disadvantages to using this language of pseudomaturity, which is rooted in assumptions about normal child development and in/authentic indicators of this, the primary focus on what follows is concerned with evidence to support or refute the contention that bereaved young people 'grow up' faster than their contemporaries, in terms of their movement across key markers of transitions to adulthood. There are also issues considered here about features of young people's behaviour that may be considered by others to be problematic.

In what follows, we are not attempting to reach definitive conclusions in the context of the contradictory nature of much of the evidence. Instead we will seek to identify some of the key issues that have been addressed in this literature, again seeking to map some of the contours of our knowledge in this area, along with some of the associated disputes as to what conclusions may be reached on the basis of what is 'known' about the outcomes of bereavement *per se* for the life transitions of young people.

Educational achievements and employment status

The evidence regarding the relevance of parental bereavement for transitions concerning educational qualifications, school-leaving and entry into labour markets is both contradictory and complex, with interactions apparent at times in relation to gender and also social class.

Only a few studies have considered employment issues, but Maclean and Wadsworth (1988) report that, by age 36, men were more likely to be unemployed and not seeking work if their parent died when they were aged under 16, than if their parents either remained together or divorced, and this group of parentally bereaved men also had a greater likelihood of earning low incomes.

Among the large-scale longitudinal UK cohort studies, Kiernan (1992), using NCDS data, found no statistically significant general relationship between parental bereavement and *early exit from the educational system*. However, Sweeting *et al.* (1998), using Scottish data, found that young men whose parent had died were the most likely of all groups to obtain *school qualifications*, but they then did not carry on into higher education. Some similar patterns of *relatively higher* educational achievements have also been found in some other studies, at least for some sub-groups of parentally bereaved children (Gregory 1965 cited by Amato 1993; Wadsworth 1991, and see Neville's and Brian's case studies in Chapter 3). Holland (2001) found that, among an opportunistic sample of adults who had been bereaved as children, 1 in 25 reported an increased focus on their academic work, while 1 in 16 had experienced a decline in academic attainment.

Based on reports from a self-selecting sample of white parents of English school pupils bereaved of a parent or sibling, Abdelnoor and Hollins (2004) found these children were significantly under-achieving in terms of qualifications at age 16, by comparison with matched controls, and parentally bereaved young people were also found to have higher anxiety scores. The authors conclude that 'the effect of bereavement may be prolonged and ... intermittent support could be needed throughout secondary and perhaps into tertiary education' (p. 52).

Nevertheless, this study and many others reveal complex patterns in the findings. Such complexity can be exemplified by the analysis of NCDS data undertaken by Elliot *et al.* (1993), in which information obtained for children at the age of 7 was compared with information for the same children at 16, dividing the children into three groups with regard to events that had taken place during those years:

1   parents were together at both ages;
2   one parent died between 7 and 16;
3   parents divorced between 7 and 16.

On maths scores, all three groups were similar at age 7, but at age 16 the group who had experienced parental death were intermediate between the other two, with the children whose parents had divorced doing worst. On reading scores, however, the pattern was different, with the children who had experienced parental death and those whose parents had divorced *both* having lower scores than the children whose parents were together. What was also striking is that this was true at age 7 *as well as* at age 16, even though all these children were living with both their parents at age 7, indicating that there was something going on in these families *prior* to the death or divorce of their parents. This resonates with the finding of Douglas *et al.* (1968: 97), using 1946 cohort data, that there was a significant association between poor educational outcomes and death of a father *if* this was preceded by a long illness.

By age 23, however, Elliott *et al.* found that the patterns had shifted again, such that the children whose parent had died seemed less adversely affected than children whose parents had divorced on all measures. Although some effect was apparent in relation to qualifications for children whose parent had died, it did not reach statistical significance.

In the analyses of the 1946 UK cohort undertaken by Maclean and Kuh (1991) at age 26, complex patterns are apparent concerning the interactions between household structure, gender, social class and educational achievements. At a general level, these authors conclude that parental divorce has a greater effect on educational attainment than parental death within this data set. However, where patterns are complex through the interaction of several variables, the numbers available in any particular group may be too small for statistical testing. For example, their data show that *non-manual women* whose parent had died were the least likely of any to go to university, but also the least likely to leave school without any qualifications, but the numbers in this sub-group were small. A statistically significant association was, however, found in relation to the educational attainments of *women from manual families* whose parent had died when compared with such women still living with both their parents. For this sub-group, the pattern of educational attainment for those whose parent had died was much more like the pattern for those whose parents had divorced or separated.

Further complexities in some of the other analyses include the presence or otherwise of siblings (Wadsworth 1991), whether or not the widowed parent re-marries (Maclean and Wadsworth 1988 citing Wadsworth and Maclean 1986), whether or not the surviving parent is in work and whether or not household income falls as a result of the death (Abelnoor and Hollins 2004).

In the context of smaller-scale, more psychologically-oriented studies, Fleming and Balmer (1996) suggest that it is unclear whether bereavement leads to a decline in school grades. Self-reports from sibling bereaved adolescents have shown a decline in several studies (Balk 1995), but a study of recorded school grades did not substantiate this pattern (Fleming and Balmer 1996).

Worden (1996) reported that 20 per cent of the parentally bereaved children and young people in his study had problems with their *learning and/ or concentration at school* during the first four months after the death. At the first anniversary of the death, 16 per cent of the bereaved children were having difficulties concentrating, compared to 6 per cent of the control group children, but at this point in time the bereaved children were not showing any greater indications of learning difficulties than the control group.

In his studies of bereavement in schools in the Humberside region of the UK, Holland (2001) found that 30 per cent of schools reported a significant loss of concentration or deterioration in schoolwork among bereaved children. Other studies have reported a significant impairment of school performance among bereaved children one year after the death of a parent (Van Eerdewegh *et al.* 1982), and less attentiveness among bereaved children than among classroom controls as rated by their teachers (Dowdney *et al.* 1999 discussed by Dowdney 2000). Children who are showing greater levels of affective distress out of school are also more likely to experience poorer school performance (Silverman and Worden 1992 discussed by Dowdney 2000). Dowdney (2000: 822) is led to the conclusion that:

> Standardised measures of attainment have been infrequently employed. Combined with child differences in academic skills, competence, and response to parental death, these limitations mean that we can only conclude that outcomes [regarding social and educational adjustment] will vary between children. Risk and protective factors, which singly or in combination may contribute to this heterogeneity, have not been the focus of these studies.

Leaving home early

Kiernan (1992), using NCDS data, conducted a focused analysis of the implications of parental bereavement for a range of possible markers of transitions in the lives of young people. In this study, leaving home early was found to be the only outcome that showed a statistically significant association with earlier parental bereavement.

Early sexual activities and partnering

The study by Kiernan (1992) did not, however, find any evidence that loss of a parent through death was associated with early partnering, sexual activities or parenthood. This contrasts markedly with the finding from a Scottish study that girls whose parent had died were the most likely of all groups to be engaged in early sexual activities and early pregnancy, even when material circumstances were taken into consideration in the analysis: 'after accounting for material deprivation, the odds of pregnancy by age 18 among the females in [the parentally bereaved] group were over eight times those who had been living with both birth parents' (Sweeting *et al.* 1998: 35).

Douglas's older study (1970) also found, in relation to the 1946 UK cohort, that the highest rates of illegitimate births among girls under 21 occurred among those who had lost a parent through death. The changing language of 'illegitimacy' (and associated social context) for births to young women outside of marriage raises the issue, however, of how we are to interpret any such data (which may vary also over time) – as a sign of deviant female behaviour, or as an early transition to adult status?

Additionally, the question of early partnering is one of the areas where contradictory tendencies have been found between different individuals. Citing the work of Hepworth *et al.* (1984) in support, Tyson-Rawson (1996) found in her smaller, in-depth study that paternally bereaved adolescent women tended to polarize, either moving quickly into committed relationships or avoiding them altogether.

Taking a somewhat longer time frame based on the UK cohort data, other studies have found higher rates of divorce and separation among adult women who were parentally bereaved as children (Wadsworth 1984 cited by Maclean and Kuh 1991; Maclean and Wadsworth 1991). These latter authors speculate that 'Women whose fathers died may try to replace their fathers by marriage, which, in turn, may lead to greater marital instability in later years when their husbands fail to match up to the idealized father image' (p. 171). Other research and clinical reports also suggest anxiety and fear about close relationships among adult women who lost a parent through death during childhood (Raphael 1984; Mireault *et al.* 2001).

Disruptive and criminal behaviours

Various studies have considered whether bereavement is associated with behaviours that are deviant or disruptive in some other way. Sweeting *et al.* (1998), for example, found that teenage women whose parents had died were more likely than any other group examined in their study to be engaging in poor *health behaviours* (smoking, drinking, drugs). And the clinical literature suggests that such behaviours may be found among bereaved young people of either sex (Raphael 1984; and see discussion in Brown 2002).

Suggestions are sometimes made that 'disruptive behaviours' or 'conduct disorders' may be a form of 'externalizing' behaviour (or 'acting out'), and may sometimes be replaced (or supplemented) by 'internalizing' behaviour, such as depression. It is important here to distinguish between behaviour that is considered aggressive or disruptive in some way, and behaviour that is defined as criminal. As with many of the other outcomes considered in this chapter, there are numerous methodological and theoretical differences regarding these topics, which may be studied from a great variety of disciplinary perspectives, ranging from labelling theory within criminology, to views of disruptive or delinquent behaviour as indicative of a 'conduct' or 'mental health' disorder. Given the ubiquity of juvenile offending, delinquency and anti-social behaviour among young people generally (apparent from self-report studies), there are major issues about how known criminal offenders come to be identified. In the context of researching bereavement, studies vary not least with regard to the exact nature of the outcome being considered, which is not always spelt out and clearly differentiated between different studies. This in turn raises issues about how far what is at issue may be a matter of law-breaking or of conflicting cultural and moral values. The behaviours in this research may thus range from angry or aggressive behaviours as identified by relevant adults, to anonymous self-reports of illegal activities in studies of cross-sections of young people as a whole, to samples of young people convicted of various offences within the formal legal system.

Focusing on *disruptive behaviour*, several studies have found no evidence of a link between parental death and 'conduct disorders' (Gersten *et al.* 1991), 'acting out behaviours' (Tyson-Rawson 1996), or 'anti-social behaviour' (Rutter *et al.* 1998). In the opposite direction, however, Elliott *et al.* (1993) did find evidence of higher levels of disruptive behaviour among parentally bereaved 16-year-olds. Worden's (1996) community-based study of parentally bereaved children and young people also found higher levels of *aggression* among bereaved children at one year after the death, as well as clear associations between bereavement and *delinquent behaviour*, especially among teenage girls whose mothers had died: 'These types of problem behaviours are correlated with high levels of parental stress and depression, along with the parent's use of less effective coping strategies, low family cohesion, more younger children, high levels of family change, and few financial resources' (1996: 64).[4]

In relation to *criminal behaviour*, the inherent processes of social selection and associated methodological weaknesses of studies that rely on official records of criminality have been noted by Loeber and Dishion (1983). The possibilities of self-fulfilling prophecies in the troubled lives of some young people from 'broken homes' have been noted by several writers (e.g. McCord 1990; Wells and Rankin 1991). McCord also points to the possibility that any links found between family structure and delinquency may be the result of them both being dependent variables of urban deprivation, and may also be mediated by other aspects of family relationships to do with 'the quality of home life rather than the number of parents' (McCord 1982: 124) (and see also, e.g. Loeber and Dishion 1983; Patterson *et al.* 1989). (We discuss such additional complexities at greater length below in relation to all outcomes.)

Nevertheless, with respect to studies of young people who have been formally convicted of offences, there has been a long history of research (dating back to the 1920s) that has considered whether or not there may be a

---

[4] However, Worden's discussion does not appear to be entirely consistent on this topic, and the patterns seem complex. It may be that this behaviour had declined by the second anniversary of the death, or that the patterns vary with age. In the discussion of delinquent adolescent girls he does not report comparisons with the control group, and later in his report he states that the research did *not* find higher levels of anger or delinquency among the bereaved adolescents compared to the control group. Yet again, when discussing bereaved children by comparison with children whose parents have divorced, he states that children whose parent had died in early adolescence, like those from divorced families, did show more aggression than older or younger children when studied at the second anniversary, and these levels were higher than in the control group.

link between 'broken homes' and 'delinquency' (McCord 1982). However, not only is this literature very confusing and uncertain about what conclusions can be drawn on this topic as a whole (Loeber and Dishion 1983), but it is also particularly confusing about the significance of homes 'broken' by parental death as one aspect of this body of work. Some studies specifically exclude this family circumstance, while others include it in an undifferentiated way within the overall category of 'broken homes'. Loeber and Dishion (1983), for example, in a major review of the quantitative literature, conclude that 'separation from parents' ranked seventh in the variety of measures they examined for effectiveness in predicting male delinquency from an early age. However, the studies on which this conclusion was based comprise some that include parental death and others that exclude this experience. Only rarely in this literature is a concerted attempt made to consider parental death as an issue in its own right.

Other writers, too, have (inadvertently) contributed to this confusion. Wadsworth is quite widely cited as having found evidence for a link between delinquency (defined by official records) and broken homes, based on his analysis of the 1946 UK cohort data. In the conclusions (1979: 115) he states that 'disruption of parent-child relationship in early life, through parental death, divorce or separation, was associated with later delinquency, and chiefly with the most unacceptable kinds of offences'. In the detailed discussion, however, it was boys from homes 'broken' by divorce or separation that were concerned in this finding.[5] Using the same data base, Douglas *et al.* (1968) conclude that there was no association between delinquency and death of a parent, and this is similar to the findings of West and Farrington (1973) (studying samples of boys from two London schools), though in their study there was a somewhat higher rate of delinquency among bereaved boys than among boys from intact families.

In Farrington's (1996) review of the literature on youth offending, the different types of 'broken home' are not always distinguished in the studies that he discusses, but where the cause of the break is considered, parental death generally appears not to be significant for offending behaviour. By contrast, Wells and Rankin (1991), in their review and meta-analysis of a great range of such studies, conclude that *both* delinquency and divorce/separation on the one hand, and delinquency and parental death on the other, show similar levels of being associated variables.

Using a different methodological approach, among those working in the

---

[5] The breakdown of figures shows that 85.8 per cent of those boys from intact homes were *not* recorded as delinquents, compared with 85.6 per cent whose fathers had died, 80.9 per cent whose mothers had died, and 73.4 per cent whose parents had divorced or separated.

criminal justice system with young offenders, bereavement also has a long history of being identified as a background feature of criminal behaviour. Shoor and Speed (1963) reported case studies, drawn from a group of 14 delinquent adolescents from one probation department in California, who were referred for clinical assessment, and found in every case, that the delinquent behaviour, either immediately or delayed, followed the death of a close loved one. Also in the USA, Gregory (1965, cited by Ayers *et al.* 2003) found that rates of delinquency were much higher among paternally bereaved young people than among those who had been bereaved of their mothers.

In the UK, Finlay and Jones (2000) studied a small group of self-selecting young offenders who chose to attend a bereavement programme. They concluded that unresolved grief for these young offenders, resulting from a variety of bereavements, could be putting them at risk of further offending (through their reliance on drugs to deal with feelings of grief) and at risk of suicide attempts. Renn (2000) offers a case study example of a persistent adult offender who was offered a series of counselling sessions, which led the therapist to identify a suppressed experience of childhood bereavement of a close friend as a significant factor in his alcohol abuse and offending behaviour. Other professionals working with youth offenders have similarly suggested that earlier bereavement and loss experiences may be significant for criminal behaviour, but such events may be overlooked by all those concerned (Youth Justice Trust 2003a, 2003b). Indeed, some youth offending teams listed bereavement as one of the five most common health issues that came to their attention (Youth Justice Trust 2001).

In a randomly selected sample of young offenders in particular areas of northern England, the Youth Justice Trust (2003c) found that almost 9 per cent had experienced the death of a parent. Boswell (1996a, 1996b) studied a specific group of young people in the UK, sentenced for particularly serious offences (constituting about 9 per cent of convicted young people in custody in 1994), and found that 10 per cent had experienced the death of a parent (a higher figure than one might expect in terms of general prevalence rates – see Chapter 1). Again, however, this is aggregated with other forms of loss (such as loss of contact) when the overall key finding is stated to be that: '57% had experienced significant loss via bereavement or cessation of contact [with "someone important"] and in some cases both' (1996: 26).

Liddle *et al.* (2002) point to the presence of clusters of risk factors in some young offenders' lives. They report, on the basis of a study of 41 persistent young offenders in one London borough, that 22 per cent had suffered (unspecified) bereavement. Similarly, Allen *et al.* (2003) found bereavement to be a relevant issue in the life histories of serious drug offenders, and suggest a need for services for such young people that are accessibly located within areas of deprivation.

Such studies need to be contextualized by a consideration of what we know about the general prevalence rates for bereavement (whether of parents or others considered to be 'significant' or 'close'), as discussed in Chapter 1. The omission of such discussion represents a serious caveat to the conclusions reached. On the other hand, many of these latter studies depend on case file records, which may under-record young people's experiences of bereavement:

> ... it was also apparent that information which was later of relevance to the work being undertaken with children and young people was not necessarily known at the outset. Where this information concerned emotional well-being, this may not be surprising given that many people need time and a degree of trust to be able to talk about experience which has had an emotional impact.
>
> (Youth Justice Trust 2003c: 20)

Overall, then, these literatures on criminality and bereavement point to some suggestive, if contradictory and inconsistent, findings (Lutzke *et al.* 1997), but are often seriously flawed by methodological difficulties. We turn next to reconsider methodological issues overall in these studies of bereavement as a 'risk' factor, that might help to account for some of the contradictions apparent in these findings so far.

Methodological considerations

Earlier in this chapter, we outlined some of the overarching methodological and theoretical issues that arise in relation to quantitative studies of 'risk' in individuals' lives over time. All research designs (whether quantitative or qualitative) involve caveats about their adequacy, with different approaches offering different strengths and limitations. Some researchers therefore explicitly offer a discussion of the limitations of their particular study, but not all writers draw our attention to such issues, so it is left to the readers to consider the adequacy of the research methodology for themselves.

A frequent criticism made of psychological studies is that they pay insufficient attention to the nature of their samples. In relation to the studies of mental health issues, discussed above, problematic issues about the samples being researched are very prevalent, and differences in the characteristics of the samples may in itself help to explain some of the contradictory findings apparent in the literature. Many studies do not even provide information about the social characteristics of the samples investigated, for example, in terms of material circumstances, social class, educational qualifications etc., and they often rely on highly contingent sampling procedures, such as volunteer or opportunistic samples based on college student populations. Christ

(2000) suggests that most samples in fact include predominantly intact middle-class families, whose resources may enable children to cope better with their bereavement experiences than those living in more difficult circumstances.

There are also significant methodological variations between studies, for example, with regard to the ways in which key concepts are operationalized and measured, with potentially substantial implications for the conclusions drawn. Worden and Silverman (1996 cited by Lowton and Higginson 2002) note the variety of different measures that are used to assess psychological problems, leading to a lack of standardized assessments as a basis for comparability across studies: 'The contentious nature of some findings, for example depression, may therefore not be due to the actual attributes of the child or the nature of their social environment, but rather due to the tools that are used'.

Several studies also point to lower levels of measured distress if the surviving parents, rather than children themselves, are asked to report on children's experiences (Dowdney 2000), although Fleming and Balmer refer to the difficulties of relying on 'the reports of grief-stricken mothers' (1996: 148) in researching adolescent bereavement responses. Other writers also discuss differences (of various kinds) in adolescent symptomatology and reports of bereavement and stressful events generally, according to whether it is the adolescents or their mothers or guardians who are asked (Thompson *et al.* 1998; Seiffge-Krenke 2000). Worden (1996) found that discrepancies of perception, in terms of how closely the parent's report of the child coincided with the child's own report, were in themselves implicated in the consequences of parental bereavement. Larger discrepancies were associated with depression in the parent, and also with sudden deaths, and children in these families were also found to be more anxious.

It is perhaps not surprising, then, that firm conclusions about any of the various health outcomes that have been considered are elusive, given such methodological complexities and frequent weaknesses in research design, such concerns being particularly relevant to the literature concerning sibling bereavement (Dowdney 2000). Many of the studies that examine 'risk' through the use of longitudinal cohort data raise even greater methodological difficulties, however. The first, and probably most important, issue to consider in relation to analyses of such data sets in terms of bereavement as a risk factor, is that – with only isolated exceptions (such as Mack 2001) – they are not trying to answer questions about bereavement experiences as such, but are instead focused on questions about divorce.

Studies that have considered experiences of family disruption in relation to outcomes in later life have developed at a rapid rate over recent years, but they have been driven by questions arising in the context of increasing divorce rates and public and policy discussions about whether divorce is seen to have deleterious long-term consequences for children. This was the case for studies that were undertaken even before the major rise in divorce rates that occurred in the last decades of the twentieth century (in the UK and other western societies). However, the language, concepts and analytic categories used in the research studies has noticeably shifted over these decades, with the earlier studies tending to consider children whose parent had been 'lost' through divorce in the same category as children whose parent had been 'lost' through death, under the general heading of 'broken families' – although this term may itself be used in highly variable ways by different researchers, or even by the same researcher at different times.[6] This concept has now been largely replaced by the concept of the 'lone parent household' – although this, too, is a category that can obscure a great deal of variability in terms of current relationships, and routes into and out of the status of 'lone parenthood'.

Where these studies have included a comparative analysis of children who have been bereaved through the death of one of their parents, this analysis has been undertaken in order to see what further light might be shed on the discussion about the effects of divorce/separation. The investigation and discussion of these data are thus very heavily framed by reference to questions that are not directly about bereavement experiences at all. Furthermore, bereavement itself is predominantly only considered by reference to one, limited, form of bereavement, namely that of one of the child's biological parents. For example: 'The fourth broad aim of our analysis was to compare parental divorce and death ... By comparing how each may be associated with the development of children *we may better understand why divorce* has such negative effects for children and so, in turn, provide better ways of ameliorating these' (Elliott *et al.* 1993: 2, emphasis added).

---

[6] Such variabilities can be found, for example, in the various publications by Wadsworth (1979, 1991; Maclean and Wadsworth 1988, 1991; Wadsworth 1984 cited by Maclean and Kuh 1991; Wadsworth and Maclean 1986) who sometimes present data separately for children whose homes have been 'broken' by divorce and by death, and sometimes present such data together, without any specific discussion of the implications for the consistency of the findings across such different analyses. There are also highly variable treatments of the implications of the re-marriage or re-partnering of the surviving or divorced parent. Thus McCord (1990) uses the concept of 'broken home' to refer to reconstituted families in conjunction with father alone households, and uses the concept of 'mother alone' to cover all cases of father absence. Later studies again, such as Hetherington (1999), specifically exclude single parent families and reconstituted households that result from the death of a parent. A focus on current household structure may also obscure considerable variations in individual histories, for example, if a child who has lost a parent through death is currently living in a (re-constituted) two-adult household.

It is thus apparent that the data are only examined in so far as they shed light on the issues of divorce. Questions that might be raised if bereavement itself were the focus of enquiry in its own right are not pursued. Similarly, while these studies have often been concerned to pay meticulous attention to exploring the meaning of inconsistencies and contradictions between different analyses in the context of the findings about divorce/separation of parents, they have not been concerned to pay similar attention to such complexities in the data in relation to the death of a parent.

It is important to note that we ourselves have not attempted here to review this literature regarding the implications of divorce/separation for children's well-being (which has already been undertaken by others, e.g. Amato 1993, 2000; Rodgers and Pryor 1998). In effect, however, what we have done is to explore this literature with a different question in mind, which centralizes the issues on the loss of a parent through death rather than the loss of a parent due to divorce or separation, reversing the lens generally used to consider this data.

As mentioned earlier, these large-scale analyses and data sets have also been the subject of extended methodological critiques concerning, for example, the adequacy of the data sets and the samples, especially in the light of differential attrition rates over time between those with varying difficulties in their lives; the validity of the information when both independent and dependent variables are measured on the basis of a single individual's responses; the adequacy of the statistical analyses, including whether multivariate analysis is used to control for other variables such as material circumstances; and how we are to infer the direction of causality on the basis of statistical associations (e.g. see the issues raised by Amato 1993; Buchanan and Ten Brinke 1997; Rogers and Pryor 1998; Sweeting *et al.* 1998). We will not reiterate these debates, but one particularly relevant issue to consider in the present context is that some of these data sets do not include sufficient numbers of bereaved individual respondents to be able to undertake the multivariate analyses that would be needed to unravel the issues concerning the death of a parent. Sweeting *et al.* (1998: 26), for example, comment that 'Low numbers in the "step"-parent and parental death categories ... mean that despite in some cases quite large differences, few of the analyses employing family structure and reason for family disruption reach a statistically significant level'. A further issue, that is particular to our current focus, is that households where a mother has died may be particularly likely to fail to respond to such surveys (Gersten *et al.* 1991).

The strength of these studies, however, rests on the fact that many of the longitudinal studies derive considerable advantages in having followed the same individuals over decades, providing reasonably strong grounds for deriving causal explanations with regard to processes over time. The direction of causality between related variables may not be altogether straightforward to establish even with longitudinal data sets, however. For example, how far do measures of parental behaviour shape, or themselves reflect, measures of children's behaviour? Where 'family time' (i.e. time parents and children spend together) has been found to be significantly related to 'outcome' measures such as offending behaviour, for example, this could suggest that children become offenders because they get less parental attention, *or* that parents want to spend less time with children who are difficult to be with and who later go on to become offenders, *or* there could be a reciprocal causality going on here over time. Sweeting *et al.* (1998) thus suggest the need to consider the processes of family lives (e.g. in terms of shared time, or levels of conflict), as well as the structures of households, in any consideration of 'outcomes'.

However, inevitably, at the same time these data sets are now often seen as rather outdated in terms of their applicability to an understanding of the lives of contemporary young people, precisely because they have taken a long time perspective. As Wadsworth comments, in relation to the study of the 1946 cohort, 'children brought up at earlier times will have a different start in life, with different consequences for adult life, compared with those born recently' (1991: 199). Several writers comment that the implications of divorce or separation may be different for more recent cohorts of children since such events have become more common and thus may be less stigmatizing (e.g. Smart 2003). But it is not clear what implications any change in the experience of divorce among different generations in itself – if true – might have for bereaved children. Loss of a parent through death may have become less likely at an absolute level, but it may also be less likely to have occurred at a relative level too, increasing the likelihood for a child of feeling a sense of difference.[7]

One particularly pertinent issue here may be the data apparent in various qualitative studies that have focused on bereaved children and young people specifically, which, as we saw above and in Chapter 3, have found that the 'effects' of the bereavement on various measures of mental health and well-being may occur in quite opposite directions for different individuals. This could have implications for the large-scale longitudinal studies where such data is aggregated, with the consequence that the different individual 'effects' cancel each other out, thus failing to show up at all in the statistical analyses. Indeed, this is one way in which qualitative data may generally help illuminate puzzles that occur with more quantitative studies, by identifying unobserved heterogeneity in the quantitative data (Kelle 2005). A related issue

---

[7] But see Chapter 1 for discussion about how this might vary between different localities.

concerns the ways in which different variables may interact in ways that may at times serve to 'mask' otherwise important associations.

In the context of research on divorce, a further methodological consideration, in relation to studies that do seem to show that divorce is related to disadvantageous outcomes, is the *extent* to which this can be said to explain or predict such outcomes, which may wane into practical insignificance in the light of the amount of variability that is left unexplained. In other words, it is not possible to explain the amount of *intra*-group variability that occurs, since there is far more variation among children still living in intact families, or among children living in similarly divorced families, than there is variability *between* these two groups. One highly eminent researcher in the area of divorce and children, Joan Kelly (2003), argues that we should stop looking at differences between children of divorced and married parents altogether, because this draws our attention away from the similarities.

For all these reasons, then, many of the more sophisticated multivariate analyses of the implications of divorce/separation try to move beyond investigations based solely on simple associations found between outcomes and household residency at a single point in time, to consider more dynamic family processes over time. More recent quantitative work (e.g. Schoon and Parsons 2002) has become considerably more sophisticated in this regard, along with associated theoretical models (Amato 2000). McCord (1990: 130), for example, looked at issues concerned with parenting and family conflict as well as household structures, and concluded in relation to the multivariate models tested (using very longitudinal data from the USA concerning delinquency among males): 'These models suggest that child-rearing differences related to the parents' behaviour have greater effects than do differences in family structure'.

More recent studies also focus on what may enable some children to live with household disruption more easily than others, using the concept of 'resilience' alongside that of 'risk' (e.g. Hetherington 1999, 2003). Resilience is demonstrated where children have 'retained competence despite the presence of adverse circumstances, in which adversity takes the form of biological, psychological, or societal shortcomings' (Garmezy 1994: 11). Various writers have expressed concerns about the concept of 'resilience', whether it is being discussed in general terms (Sanford 1991 cited by Atwool 1997), or in relation to bereavement issues specifically: 'Neither the children nor the surviving parent will bounce back to the way they were before the death, as resilience implies. Rather, both must transform their relationship to the parent/spouse who dies and work to build a life that incorporates the painful reality of the loss' (Christ 2000: 242).

In more general terms, Garmezy suggests that the concept of 'resilience' runs the risk of promoting the myth that individuals can overcome adversities if they just put in the right effort, although Atwool (1997) points out that resilience is not an isolated individual characteristic, but a feature of individual, family and social characteristics, and their complex inter-relationships (issues to which we will return towards the end of this chapter).

Such complexities mean that the generalizations derived from quantitative studies cannot be used in any simple way to extrapolate to individual biographies: 'There is no inevitable path down which children who experience these events [of family disruption] will travel' (Burghes 1994 quoted by Sweeting *et al.* 1998: 17). Indeed, in the context of a lifetime of work on longitudinal data sets in the USA, Hetherington (2003: 217) has recently commented: 'When I began studying divorce, like most investigators I had a pathogenic model of divorce ... Now, after 35 years of studying divorced families, what impresses me is not the inevitability of adverse outcomes, but the diversity of adjustment in parents and children in response to marital dissolution'.

Taken overall, however, such quantitative studies of divorce have had a powerful impact on policy and public debates. But, in the light of the primary focus of such studies on questions regarding divorce/separation, it is perhaps not surprising that evidence regarding the significance of the death of a parent for later outcomes may sometimes be subject to simplistic generalizations. Death of a parent may thus be described as occupying an intermediate position, between the positive benefits of living in an intact family and the negative effects of living with a divorced or remarried parent, in relation to the likelihood of undesirable outcomes for the children concerned. As Rodgers and Pryor (1998) comment in relation to the dangers of presenting misleading simplifications of the data concerning divorce/separation, it is all to easy for such generalizations to gain the status of a kind of lay or mythological 'expert' truth.

Even in Amato's careful and painstaking systematic review of this literature on parental divorce/separation, we find parental death discussed in simplified terms, because his focus of interest is what may be concluded about the implications of divorce/separation for children: 'Most studies show that well-being is lowest in divorced families, intermediate in bereaved families, and highest in intact families ... This suggests that although the loss of a parent through death is problematic, an additional factor is involved in divorce that further lowers the well-being of some children' (Amato 1993: 27).

Rodgers and Pryor (1998: 40), despite their concern, noted above, not to oversimplify the evidence concerning divorce/separation, state even more categorically than Amato in relation to the death of a parent:

> The overriding impression from studies of bereavement is that neither loss nor absence are of great importance. Parental death clearly does not lead to the same range and degree of adverse outcomes as separation. The areas that do show associations may well reflect the

acute effect of the experience of loss eg bedwetting in childhood, or the consequence of reduced supervision, as with substance use in the teenage years. These problems do not appear to have a serious lasting impact.

A rather more circumspect conclusion is given be Elliott *et al.* (1993: 12): 'Two broad conclusions can be drawn from these results: that overall, parental divorce has more negative consequences for children's behaviour and educational attainment than the death of a parent, but that patterns vary a good deal depending on which aspect of children's behaviour is examined'.

Similarly, while Buchanan and Ten Brinke (1997) write about a 'gradient' of risk with regard to psychological problems in adult life – with membership of a lone-widow(er) household at 16 years of age being in the middle of the gradient – they also highlight the significance of being in care or severely disadvantaged in childhood as being more important than any variation in the structure of the childhood family/household.

Whatever conclusions one draws from the evidence with regard to the consequences of *divorce*, in relation to furthering our understanding of the significance for children of *death* of a parent, the generalization that death is somehow 'intermediate' in its effect (between intact families and divorced/separated families) is likely to be both unhelpful and oversimplified. Amato himself goes on to demonstrate, in his reviews (1993, 2000) of the evidence about divorce/separation, that it is an extremely complex matter to tease out what are the relevant individualized processes that may underlie any statistical associations. Bereavement is not given the same detailed attention because it is not the focus of concern, but it is possible, maybe even likely, that a more careful consideration of the evidence on bereavement will show that the picture is far more complex than these statements would lead us to expect. Contrast the statements above from Amato, and Rodgers and Pryor, for example, with the following conclusions reached by one recent quantitative analysis of a large-scale data set of the lives of Scottish teenagers: 'those (males) whose parents had separated [were] the most likely *and those who had experienced the death of a parent least likely* to have no school qualifications ... [among females], the opposite is true. The *highest* rates of smoking, drinking, experience of drugs, early heterosexual intercourse and pregnancy occurred *among those whose parents had died*' (Sweeting *et al.* 1998: 39, emphasis added). Perhaps the most pressing task facing researchers into bereavement as a 'risk' factor in the lives of children and young people, then, is to consider the evidence in a more complex way.

Exploring complexities

One of the difficulties in reaching clear and unequivocal conclusions from these studies, then, is that it is difficult to establish the (objective) complexities, (subjective) meanings and subtleties of the lives of individual children by reference to large-scale quantitative data that has perforce to rely on approximate operationalizations of what may be considered relevant indicators of family and life experiences.

More recent quantitative studies of divorce and separation, and of adversity more generally, have sought to develop more sophisticated statistical analyses to unravel some of the complexities and contradictions found in earlier studies of outcomes for children and young people, regarding concepts of both risk and resilience (Haggerty 1994; Amato 2000). Such analyses do not generally seem to have been considered for children and young people who have experienced (parental) bereavement. Nevertheless, there may be some useful food for thought about the issues for bereaved children and young people which can be gleaned from these more advanced quantitative investigations of the consequences of divorce/separation. There are a number of issues that have been identified as influential in relation to the experience of divorce/separation for children, and that are likely to be (and in some cases, have been established to be) relevant to the experiences of bereaved children. These findings can also be considered alongside medical and psychological research studies of bereaved children and young people themselves, where these have considered such further complexities.

A variety of cross-cutting and contextual variables may thus underlie some of the complexities and puzzles in the findings discussed above. These may be understood by reference to individual differences, family relationships, aspects of social structure and the clustering of certain experiences in processes over time.

Individual differences

We have suggested throughout this book so far that the significance of a particular category of bereavement may depend very much on the meaning the death has for the individual concerned. In understanding statistical patterns in large data sets, it is difficult to take account of how young people themselves frame and understand a bereavement, but this factor may help to account for the ways in which opposite changes seem to occur between different bereaved individuals. For example, religious beliefs may both shape, and be shaped by, bereavement experiences (Hogan and DeSantis 1994), although here again the evidence is complex (Balk 1991a; Ringler and Hayden 2000). Thus Holland comments that 'The outcomes for [the adult interviewees giving retrospective accounts of childhood bereavement] were sometimes quite different in similar circumstances' (2001: 135).

Rodgers and Pryor (1998) conclude, in relation to divorce/separation, that it is likely that *within* one family, individual children may show contradictory outcomes, and this is very likely to be relevant to bereaved families also – although in neither context has this been directly investigated through quantitative data. Balmer (reported in Fleming and Balmer 1996) suggests the possibility of *personality factors* affecting the individual's adjustment to loss. While many/most bereaved adolescents may show resilience and the possibilities of increased maturity through crisis, she suggests that there may be a minority who are at risk of longer-term negative outcomes.

Seiffge-Krenke (2000), in a more general exploration of causal links between stressful events (including death of a relative), adolescent symptomatology and individual coping style, found that coping style was more important than the type of stressor for predicting (in terms of statistical modelling) adolescent symptomatology. Age 15 was identified as a time when young people encounter 'a turning point in the use of more efficacious and adaptive strategies in dealing with stress' (2000: 677). She suggests that less effective coping styles, defined as withdrawal and avoidance, have also been found to be more common among diverse clinical samples of adolescents. But the patterns are very complex in terms of linking different stressors, coping styles and symptomatology at different ages, with early adolescents apparently more at risk because they have not yet developed effective coping strategies, and also evidence of negative feedback loops resulting in a downward spiral of effects. Furthermore, such studies of individual differences need to consider further how these may interrelate with features of social context (a point to which we return below).

Other general studies of young people and risk point to such factors as scholastic achievement and self-esteem as compensating for risk, although such variables offer only limited protection where an individual is experiencing risk factors across a variety of life domains (Gerard and Buehler 2004).

Family relationships

Relationships prior to death
The levels of conflict and other family processes that occurred between parents *prior* to divorce have been identified as important for children's functioning *after* divorce (Amato and Booth 1996 cited in Sweeting *et al.* 1998; Amato 2000; Hetherington 2003). Rodgers and Pryor (1998) similarly stress the need to view divorce and separation as a process rather than a single event. This points, perhaps, to considerations of parental relationships prior to the bereavement of a child. The evidence from Douglas *et al.* 1968 is interesting in suggesting that it was the presence or absence of long illness *prior*

to the death of a parent that was associated with poor outcomes. This study found that it was *only* when a father's death was preceded by a long illness that there was a noticeable association with educational performance. Thus, while at first glance bereavement may appear to be something closer to a single event, the possibility of preceding ill health or other difficult life circumstances is clearly relevant to processes over time.

Discussions concerning the implications of parental conflict both prior to, and continuing after, divorce or separation point to pervasive findings that parental conflict is related to children's well-being, particularly if it is expressed violently (either physically or verbally), is poorly resolved, and the child feels caught in the middle (Amato 1993, 2000; Rodgers and Pryor 1998). Sweeting *et al.* (1998) found that bereaved teenagers were as likely as separated families to have been experiencing parental conflict. This does point to a possibility that for some bereaved children, death of a parent can actually improve their life situation if it leads to a final resolution of overt parental conflict. Worden (1996) found that the pre-death relationship between a child or young person and a parent who died mediated some of the impact of the bereavement, especially the level of ambivalence.

Single-parent households

Other issues concern the nature of relationships *after* a death has occurred. There are two issues that are discussed in relation to the presence of only one parent in a household as a result of death or divorce/separation. One concerns the significance of having only one parenting adult available in a household, and the other concerns the personal resources and resilience of the surviving/resident parent.

In relation to the presence of only *one parent* in the household, Amato (1993: 27) discusses evidence that suggests that parental loss *per se* may indeed have undesirable implications for children's lives, and finds support for this view: 'The majority of studies ... [show] that both divorce and parental death are associated with lower child well-being'.

In this context, it is interesting to note the finding of Sweeting *et al.* (1998), that time spent in family activities (as reported by teenagers themselves) was strongly associated with more desirable outcomes, and also that bereaved teenagers were as likely as separated families to have less family time together (a finding replicated by Ely et al 2000). What is not clear from their data is how far this is itself related to the restrictions on leisure time that might be experienced by a single-parent household. It would therefore be interesting to be able to explore this issue in interaction with parental employment status. The earlier research by West and Farrington (1973), based on a different sample, similarly reported the significance of amount of time spent by parents with their 10-year-old sons for likelihood of delinquency.

Relationship with surviving parent
Related to the issue of lone parenthood, is the question of the quality of the relationship between *the remaining parent and the child after parental death*. In the context of divorce, the quality of the relationship between the resident divorced parent and the child has been found to be relevant to children's well-being, both prior to and after the divorce itself. McCord (1990: 132), for example, using a very long-term data set concerning males in the USA, found that 'effects of parental absence [in general terms] largely depended on the competence of the remaining parent'. Similarly, Hetherington (2003: 226) concluded from analysis of several large-scale longitudinal data sets in the USA, that 'The quality of inter-parental relationships, parent-child relationships, and to a lesser extent, those with siblings and grandparents can have a profound influence on the adjustment of children in divorced and remarried families'.

This issue may be relevant to the extent to which the death of a parent is likely to be felt as a serious bereavement by a child, but Mack (2001) found that parental death was not followed by a poorer quality relationship with the surviving parent. Christ (2000) discusses the significance of the remaining parent's ability to parent, and Gersten *et al.* (1991) also found that 'poor parenting practices' mediated the impact of parental death on children (citing Sandler *et al.* 1988 and West *et al.* 1991). Thus adult depression among those who experienced childhood parental death has been found to be lower if the surviving parent is described as warm and empathetic (Saler and Skolnick 1992). Similarly, Haine *et al.* (2006) found positive parenting constituted a protective resource in terms of parentally bereaved children's mental health, while Saldinger et al (2004) found that child-centred parenting was associated with lower levels of symptoms among bereaved children. Worden (1996) found that different children's and adolescents' relationships with their surviving parent could show quite opposite tendencies, with some becoming closer and others becoming more hostile. His study assessed 56 per cent of surviving parents as depressed four months after the death, a figure that fell to 40 per cent by the second anniversary of the death. Furthermore, a 'passive coping style' on the part of the surviving parent 'increased the likelihood of a child experiencing emotional and behavioural difficulties' (1996: 45).

The relationship with the surviving parent is likely, in turn, to reflect the *resources of the lone parent*, referring to the degree of stress experienced by the resident, divorced or bereaved parent, as well as the personal resources available to lone parents and the degree to which they may be able to adjust (Amato 1993, 2000; Lutzke *et al.* 1997). It is widely argued, for example, that widow(er)s are at risk of poor physical and mental health (Gersten *et al.* 1991; Worden 1996).

Family dynamics
Other features of *continuing family relationships* have also received attention in mediating the impact of a significant bereavement. It is clear that relationships with surviving family members can be experienced as either very problematic or very supportive after bereavement. People may, for example, strive for 'mutual protection', or may impose particular expectations on children and young people (Demi and Gilbert 1987; Worden 1996; Sutcliffe *et al*. 1998 – and we saw both these features in Neville's case study in Chapter 3). There is evidence, for example, of young people seeking to avoid thinking about the death of a sibling in order to be able to support and soothe their parents (Demi and Gilbert 1987). Balmer (reported in Fleming and Balmer 1996) found that surviving siblings were reported by sibling bereaved adolescents as being the least helpful of their family members, although Worden (1996) found that adolescents were more likely than younger children to select a sibling over the surviving parent as the family member to whom they were closest after the death of a parent. Worden also found widespread tendencies for children and adolescents to be worried about the safety of their surviving parent, and to be trying to be 'good' and helpful – a striking example of how the children and young people themselves could be active moral agents in the situation. But some family relationships may deteriorate to a point of 'extreme alienation' (Gray 1989) or outright abuse (Cross 2002).

Several studies point to the significance of the well-being and 'competence' of survivors in providing support to each other (Gray 1989; Gersten *et al*. 1991; Fleming and Balmer 1996; Worden 1996; Black 2002). Guerriero and Fleming (1985 discussed in Balk 1995) report that, where families show emotional closeness and personal communication, bereaved adolescents report a decline in feelings of fear, loneliness and numbness over time, but where there is emotional distance and little communication they report feelings of guilt and anger rather than shock or loneliness. In a later discussion, Fleming and Balmer (1996: 147) review evidence about family support, which could sometimes be conflicting, but conclude that, '[A] bereaved adolescent could view the family environment as helpful in adjusting to death if that family unit is cohesive, allows for members to express opinions, and is low in conflict'.

Tyson-Rawson, researching paternally bereaved women college students, found that several aspects of family relationships could act as mediating factors in the resolution of grief, including: the openness of communication in the family; the ability of the surviving parent and others to 'provide stability and continuity in day-to-day life' (1996: 163); and the emotional context for the expression of the distress of bereavement.

The issue of re-marriage or re-partnering of the surviving parent after a parental bereavement is mentioned as an issue in some studies, but again the evidence is confusing. Worden (1996) actually found that this seemed to reduce children's anxiety levels and concerns about the safety of the surviving parent.

In relation to studies of children and young people's adjustment to parental divorce, there is mixed evidence about the relevance of grandparents in mediating the children's experiences (Hetherington 2003; Kelly 2003), but there appears to be little research into the significance of grandparents or other relatives in mediating experiences to do with bereavement.

The complex *inter*relationships of these various processes also need more widespread consideration. In discussing the results of the national survey of children's mental health, Meltzer *et al.* (2000) (citing Tamplin *et al.* 1998) point out that children's mental disorders could impact on the rest of the family, including relationships between adults, between adults and children, and with other family members. They also found that parental behaviour could be affected, for example, in terms of smoking more.

Gender, class and race

As noted in Chapter 1, parental bereavement rates are likely to vary between different social groups, pointing to the relevance of social structure. In this regard, models of outcomes also need to take account of broad structural differences, including gender, class and race, all of which may also be manifest in relation to both family relationships and individual differences. As Marris (1996: 118) has observed, 'Inequalities of power affect both vulnerability to bereavement and the ability to recover from it'. Such inequalities of power are also socially structured or patterned in certain observable ways.

Seiffge-Krenke (2000) discusses significant *gender differences* in coping styles, stress reporting and symptomatology. One particularly relevant finding here is that of Reinherz *et al.* (1993), who suggest that the death of a parent is associated with major depression in late adolescence for girls but not for boys. In the context of childhood bereavement studies more broadly, it is clear that gender can make a considerable difference, both in terms of the child concerned and in terms of the surviving parent (Douglas 1970; Maclean and Kuh 1991; Kiernan 1992; Black 1993; Worden 1996; Sweeting *et al.* 1998). Furthermore, this interplay between gender of parent and of child may work differently for different outcomes. If the resident/surviving parent later remarries, again, the implications of living with a step-parent may differ between the child of the same sex as the step-parent and the child of opposite sex. Perhaps in line with the gender differences found in depression outcomes (discussed earlier), Balmer (1992 cited by Fleming and Balmer 1996) reports some evidence that girls may show higher levels of anxiety and sleep problems than boys after the death of a sibling, and Guerriero and Fleming (1985 discussed by Balk 1995) similarly found that girls, unlike boys, expressed an increasing sense of confusion over time after a sibling bereavement. However,

Balmer found no evidence for Raphael's assertion that boys may turn to drugs and alcohol. Tyson-Rawson (1996) (drawing on a variety of sources) suggests that girls may have more opportunities to grieve openly but may also be more expected to take on care-taking roles.

With regard to the gender of the parent who has died, there have been many suggestions over the years that it may be more disruptive of everyday life if it is the mother rather than the father who has died (Tyson-Rawson 1996; Worden 1996), and that maternal death signifies a greater risk factor than paternal death for adult outcomes such as depression (Dowdney 2000). Balmer found that sibling bereaved adolescents reported mothers as more helpful than fathers, but Hogan and Balk (both discussed in Fleming and Balmer 1996) found that fathers were closer to teenagers' own self-reports in their assessment of the teenagers' grief reactions. Worden (1996) found that, two years after the death of their mothers, adolescents living with their fathers were the least likely group to report a good relationship with their surviving parent. Difficulties in feeling 'close' to fathers during the teenage years are also widely discussed in the literature on the family lives generally of young people (see e.g. Gillies *et al.* 2001).

Some studies that have paid explicit attention to *social class* dimensions in the data sets have found this to be a significant issue in the patterns that are found between various outcomes of both divorce/separation and parental death (Lutzke *et al.* 1997). Furthermore, as noted above in relation to educational achievements, this social class effect may differ between the sexes (Maclean and Wadsworth 1991). We can also see some patterns in the data presented by Elliott *et al.* (1993) that suggest an interaction between the gender of the young person and social class, with boys from manual-class homes who lost a parent before the age of 15 showing similar patterns of malaise to boys whose parents had divorced, but this pattern was not there for girls, nor for boys from non-manual homes.

Interactions between the variables of social class and the sex of the parent who has died are particularly likely to be apparent in relation to the implications of the death of fathers for *material well-being* (Douglas *et al.* 1968; Maclean and Wadsworth 1988; Gersten *et al.* 1991; Wadsworth 1991). Elliott *et al.* (1993) found that, although financial problems in the families of 16-year-olds were more common after divorce than after death, this very clearly related to social class. For non-manual children, household income remained very stable after parental death. For skilled manual children, household income deteriorated after parental death, but only for unskilled manual children did this decline of income come close to the decline in income experienced by children from divorced families. In considering how death of a parent (since age 7) seemed to affect children less seriously than divorce of parents (since age 7), Elliott *et al.* also note that the implications of divorce were reduced once income and social class were taken into account. However, the study by Gersten *et al.* (1991) did not find depression among 8–15-year-old parentally bereaved children to be any higher among those whose material circumstances had declined as a result of the death than among those whose material circumstances remained stable.

In the Scottish data analysed by Sweeting *et al.* (1998), the bereaved families were found to be like separated families with regard to material deprivations, and this study is notable for the extent of the various outcomes that were found to be associated with bereavement (as discussed earlier). Furthermore, these findings were later replicated in another cohort study of British data (Ely et al 2000). Worden (1996: 86) found that children from more affluent families reported less sleep disturbance, concentration difficulties or learning problems after the death of a parent: 'Children from more affluent families were less likely to be in the at-risk group at any time over the two years [of the study]'.

As noted above, Amato (1993) draws attention to the limitations of those many studies of the outcomes of parental divorce/separation which do not control for changes in material circumstances. Among those which do consider such issues, some find that material resources 'explain' a good deal – but by no means all – of the variation in outcomes for children between lone-parent and two-parent households. Nevertheless, the material implications of divorce have received more attention than bereavement, primarily in terms of direct material resources, but also sometimes in terms of *subsequent disruptions*. Amato's later review (2000) thus points to changes of school or moving house as consistently related to negative outcomes for children whose parents had divorced. Here, too, however, we must be aware of the complexities, since the effects may not always be uniformly un/desirable. Amato concludes: 'it may not be the absolute number of such changes, but particular types of change, that are problematic for children' (1993: 34). Worden's (1996) study of children and young people who had experienced the death of a parent found that the number of changes in daily life mediated some of the effects of the bereavement, particularly as time progressed. By the second year, the children who reported the greatest number of changes also reported more family arguments and poorer relationships with their parent. Furthermore, the number of changes experienced by the family as a whole related to parental depression.

In their questionnaire-based study, Harrison and Harrington asked adolescents to indicate how much their lives had changed as a result of bereavements experienced. While we cannot know what changes may have lain behind the responses given, Harrison and Harrington's further analysis (2001: 162) showed that this additional factor was seen to mediate significantly the association between some categories of bereavement (parents, grandparents and aunts/uncles) and measured depression, leading them to conclude that 'the effects of this kind of loss depend to an important extent on the changes they bring about in the child's life'.

The ways in which issues of *race* may interrelate with those of class and material circumstances have not received attention within the empirical literature – not even in relation to divorce (Amato 2000). One rare exception here is the study by Thompson *et al.* (1998), which found that some measures of the effects of parental death were in fact moderated by race, with young people from minority groups showing *lower* levels of externalizing distress, according to reports by their guardians.

The discussion by Desai and Bevan (2002), however, points to the potential of important further issues in this regard. These authors draw attention to the ways in which racism may itself be centrally understood as a form of loss. Ethnic minority groups may already have experienced significant losses of various kinds in their lives, through experiences of migration, disadvantage and racism, which may increase their vulnerability when dealing with the loss of bereavement. Young people may face particular dilemmas in this regard, as they face the loss of, or disruptions to, their family and cultural histories, while themselves seeking to forge new and different identities and lifestyles from those of their parents in the countries of their birth. (And see the case study of Shirleen in Chapter 3 for a vivid illustration of some of these issues).

Multiple bereavements and problematic life events

While many of the studies discussed in this chapter have examined the significance of a single bereavement *per se* as a 'risk' factor (particularly bereavement through the death of a parent), the importance of a *constellation of issues and difficulties* in any individual's life is suggested in other studies. From this perspective, it may not be the bereavement as a single event that increases the risk of negative outcomes for the young person, but the way in which bereavement features within the individual's life course more broadly, including both antecedent and consequent events. The data available from the UK longitudinal studies, for example, has pointed to the importance of bereavement as potentially precipitating a move into state care, such that it is those bereaved children who have entered the state care system who are seen to have experienced negative outcomes (Buchanan and Ten Brinke 1997). More subtle processes and complex life events by which particular children and young people come to be especially negatively affected by bereavement have yet to be properly considered in the research, although Sandler *et al.* (1997) suggest that relatively minor additional stressful events may affect children's adjustment in the context of a single major negative life event like parental death.

Rodgers 1990 also discusses evidence of the significance of *multiple disadvantage* apparent in the lives of some individuals in the large-scale data sets (and see Carron and Rutter 1991 cited by Seiffge-Krenke 2000). Harrison and Harrington similarly conclude that a particular bereavement may be significant in the context of multiple losses (including multiple deaths) in the lives of young people, drawing on data from their community-based samples to show that young people who reported the death of a parent were also significantly more likely to report other deaths, for example, of an aunt or uncle. Furthermore, 'Adolescents who experienced four losses or more had a much higher risk of the depression category ... than adolescents who had never experienced a loss' (2001: 162).

The significance of *multiple problematic life events* (including bereavement) is also stressed by Meltzer *et al.* (2000: 102) whose analysis of the national UK survey of the mental health of children and young people found that 'The number of stressful life events does seem to have a cumulative effect on psychiatric morbidity with prevalence rates ranging from 7% among children with 1 event to 16% of those who had 3 events to 34% of children who had experienced 5 or more stressful life events'.

The community-based samples studied by Gersten *et al.* (1991: 490) also produced evidence that experiences of low levels of 'stable positive family circumstances' and 'high levels of negative life events' were important factors mediating the effects of parental death for children's depression. As discussed earlier, Worden (1996) found that the 'dysfunction' of the surviving parent (particularly in terms of a 'passive' rather than an 'active' coping style) was an important mediator of the consequences of children's experiences of parental death and 'this dysfunction ... consistently put the children at risk' (1996: 78). But this in turn tended to be associated with a variety of other difficulties, including: many family changes following on from the death; health problems in the family; financial problems; larger family size; younger age of the surviving parent; and, finally, deaths that were unexpected.

From the perspective of smaller-scale studies, MacDonald and Marsh (2001) have also commented on the striking way some individual lives seem to be blighted by multiple disadvantages, with bereavement featuring as one such issue that may substantially increase the individual's vulnerability to negative consequences of other difficult life events. Quite how such multiple difficult events may occur in the lives of particular individuals, and the nature of the underlying processes involved, is open to speculation: 'Although it is tempting to ponder the possibility that parental death increases child vulnerability to later stressors or loss, this hypothesis has never been tested' (Dowdney 2000: 823). In this respect, it may be worth noting Wadsworth's (1979) discussion of evidence suggesting that early family disruption is associated with differences in physical as well as mental reactions to stress in early adult life (in the form of lower pulse rates among boys).

The view of bereavement as a potential 'risk' factor within a more complex set of processes and events that may increase risk or enhance resilience in an individual's life is consonant with debates about how to progress psychosocial studies of development and psychopathological outcomes generally (Rutter 2000). Despite a forthright and detailed discussion of the difficulties in this research approach and the studies undertaken within this tradition, Rutter (2000: 398) remains optimistic about the possibilities for further understanding of 'environmental mediation mechanisms' if there is a revolution of methods to create 'high-quality, rigorous research'. In relation to the changes experienced in relation to divorce or separation, Rodgers and Pryor (1998: 45) suggest that 'our understanding of how short-term distress in children relates to longer-term outcomes is rudimentary', and call for studies that enable a consideration of processes in interaction over time.

Other writers in the field of risk and resilience research more generally also point to the fact that a single risk factor is unlikely in itself to precipitate serious negative consequences. Indeed, Newman (2002) suggests that a single, or moderate, difficult experience may be a source of learning as well as disadvantage. Kessler *et al.* (1997: 1101), in their wide-ranging research on childhood adversity and adult psychiatric disorder, drawing on data from the US National Comorbidity Survey, found that there was strong clustering of childhood adversities, leading them to conclude:

> ... caution is needed in interpreting the results of pervious single-adversity single-disorder studies as documenting unique effects of specific childhood adversities on specific adult disorders. Future studies need to assess a broader range of adversities and disorders and to explore the existence and effects of commonly occurring adversity clusters. Replication is needed to verify that the effects of childhood adversities are mostly on first onset rather than on the creation of vulnerabilities that lead to increased risk of persistence.

Newman (2002: 12), like others (such as Garmezy 1994), points out the significance of structural issues in this regard, such that, 'Risk factors will be intensified when the child lives in an environment where poverty, racism and low social capital are endemic'. In the area of youth development specifically, Gerard and Buehler (2004: 1844) point to the significance of multiple problems that span across different areas of an individual's life: 'youth are increasingly challenged as risk factors accumulate. Particularly harmful is an accumulation of stressors that spans across multiple contexts'. Again, however, the complexity of the issues is highlighted, since ethnic differences had varying implications for resilience: 'Although our study demonstrated cross-cutting patterns of stress resistance, evidence of ethnic differences points to the error of assuming that one model of development fits all' (2004: 1846).

Conclusions

This has been an exploratory excursion into the evidence available from the various longitudinal, psychological and medical studies that use a structured methodology to consider the significance of bereavement for experiences in the teenage and early adult years. In this chapter we have concentrated on the more established bodies of literature based on empirical research that have focused primarily on parental and (to a lesser extent) sibling bereavement in relation to a variety of possible outcomes for young people, sometimes extending into their adult lives.

In doing so, we have not discussed *other sorts of studies*, notably those which discuss whether bereavement is a factor in the development of some physical illnesses, or non-specific visits to primary health care professionals (Lloyd-Williams *et al.* 1998). Guerriero and Fleming (discussed in Balk 1995) found evidence that health problems might persist over a period of at least four years, and Worden (1996) found clear evidence of a link between physical ill health and parental bereavement among adolescents. There is some evidence from the UK longitudinal studies that ill health during childhood, and up to age 25, might be associated with parental death (Wadsworth 1991). Nevertheless, Lutzke *et al.* (1997) suggest that the evidence concerning parental bereavement and children's somatic complaints – as with many other outcomes – may be inconsistent. Other studies have particularly focused on specific aspects of physical and mental health, such as eating disorders (e.g. Shoebridge and Gowers 2000).

We have also not paid specific attention to *particular forms of death*, such as perinatal loss, neonatal loss, abortion or suicide, nor to particularly traumatic deaths, whether of close relatives or friends or others, which may be associated with post-traumatic stress disorders. There is also a small set of studies that consider bereavement following *death of a peer* (although La-Grand 1985 cited by Balk 1995 suggests that these are the forgotten grievers in terms of both research and everyday relationships) and a few studies that consider *death of a grandparent*. It has not been possible in this current project to give these additional literatures the attention they deserve,[8] although the existence of such literatures does in turn raise important issues about where we draw the lines, in terms of defining particular experiences as 'different', or as showing continuities with other experiences of loss and bereavement.

What seems to be evident from the literature that we have considered is that many of the findings are complex and equivocal, and researchers have

---

[8] References on these areas are available direct from the author: J.C.Ribbens-mccarthy@open.ac.uk.

not always been concerned with exploring and acknowledging this complexity (or even reporting it very accurately at times). At present, it is perfectly possible to draw on different studies selectively to support a variety of different arguments, depending on the point of view of the writer(s). In the longitudinal studies, particularly, research attention has been focused overwhelmingly on issues to do with divorce and separation, not with bereavement as such. Perhaps, taken overall, this review can suggest that there is indeed 'something going on' here, and that it is likely that there can be important negative (and sometimes positive) outcomes for some bereaved children – while some outcomes might, indeed, be double-edged. Such outcomes may depend on the nature of the bereavement, how the individual experiences it, and also the presence of other factors. Furthermore, as Muir Gray (2001) discusses more generally in relation to evidence-based health care, in evaluating the effectiveness of forms of care there are judgements to be made about how many studies are needed before we decide we have good evidence, and about whether or not all the studies have to agree with each other.

The 'effects' of bereavement have thus been shown – by at least some studies, in some circumstances – to carry implications for educational and learning processes and outcomes, for early home leaving, for early sexual activities and poor health behaviours, and possibly for aggressive or delinquent behaviours (although in many of these areas the literature is inconsistent and confusing). There is certainly evidence for high levels of short-term distress and depressive symptoms for large numbers – but by no means all – of young people who experience a 'significant' bereavement in their lives. And while some may demonstrate enhanced self-worth and express a sense of increased maturity as a result of bereavement experiences, others appear to be at risk of reduced self-esteem, particularly where parental death is associated with a considerable number of life changes. Furthermore, the structured methodologies of the research studies explored in this chapter are unlikely to be able to capture the ambiguities and ambivalences that may characterize any individual response to a particular bereavement.

One particularly noteworthy feature of the literature concerns the possibility – even the likelihood – that children and young people may continue to feel the consequences of a significant bereavement *over the years* of their young lives. Given Worden's finding (1996) that problems among parentally bereaved children were greater at two years than at one year after the death, Christ (2000) suggests that many studies operate within too short a time scale to really assess the impact of bereavement. The implications for adult lives are even more difficult to establish, however, but again much of the evidence we have considered in this chapter demonstrates the existence of long-term risks for some young people, especially in conjunction with other difficult issues in their lives.

The confusion and inconsistencies in much of the literature are very striking, however, and researchers themselves seem to be at a loss to know how to explain these. The primary emphasis in the literature reviewed here has been upon the particular methodology that seeks to establish 'risk' through the identification of statistically significant associations between variables, associations that are higher than would be expected among those who have not experienced bereavement. This emphasis on statistical significance means that some trends may be disregarded when they might still be relevant. It may be, for example, that numbers are too small to enable these tests to be applied. Some trends may simply fail to reach the statistically defined significance level, such that outcome variables may show 'a trend . . . that [is] not always statistically significant' (Black 1991: 137). Conversely, we also have to be careful to acknowledge that statistical significance can tell us that an association between variables is unlikely to be due to the chance effects of random sampling, but it cannot in itself be used to indicate *practical significance* with regard to policies or interventions.

Besides these statistically-based studies, in this chapter we have also drawn on other literature that is based in psychological and/or medical studies, without necessarily using such large samples. Some of this literature provides further important insights into some of the issues that may underlie the statistical patterns. One such issue is the significance of *how young people themselves frame and understand* bereavement experiences. Balk illustrates this issue by reference to the transition to senior school that is a 'normal' feature of the lives of American young people as they enter the teenage years, but which can also constitute an important experience of change and loss. Balk suggests that this experience is very much helped if it is understood as 'a regular, expected event that provides evidence of maturing' (1995: 346). Such issues of meaning and understanding may help to account for the ways in which opposite changes seem to occur between different bereaved young people (e.g. in terms of the implications of a significant bereavement for their educational outcomes). The significance of the subjective interpretations of the individual were directly considered by Mireault and Bond (1992), who found that, among college students who had experienced parental death during childhood, level of anxiety and depression was higher than with a control group, but this was significantly mediated by the students' perceptions of themselves and others as vulnerable to future loss. At a more general level, Rutter (2000) points to the crucial importance of personal meanings in his discussion of psychosocial research as a whole (discussed further in Chapter 6).

Another possibility is that there may be quite *contradictory processes* at stake depending on which outcome is considered desirable. Tyson-Rawson (1996: 162), for example, distinguishes between 'matters relating to the practical realities of life' and 'personal growth and positive outcomes'. Emotional detachment from the person who had died (in her study, this being the father) seemed to be helpful to the former, but continuing emotional attachment seemed to be helpful for the latter.

If we are to understand this more clearly we need more direction attention to bereavement issues within such longitudinal data sets, that can pay proper attention to the *complexities*, interrelationships and cross-cutting dimensions of the data, to help unravel which factors are likely to be associated with which problematic outcomes, under which circumstances of bereavement. Given the complexity of these issues, it is also important to integrate this discussion with other evidence, and for a dialogue between these longitudinal studies and those based in the medical literature. Thus, reviews of the literatures on parentally bereaved children (e.g. Tennant *et al.* 1980; Dowdney 2000) do not refer to the extensive work done around the large-scale general longitudinal studies, and these latter studies, in turn, do not refer to the medically-oriented literature. More dialogue between these various bodies of work would seem to be desirable, for both identifying the larger patterns and trying to fill in more of the complexities.

There may also be a need for the insights that may be gained from more qualitative methodologies (Chapter 3). Given the importance of the *meaning* that any particular bereavement has for the individual, studies that have to rely on the category of the relationship involved (e.g. parent, sibling etc.) can only roughly approximate the variable of 'significant bereavement'. Even with the category of parental death, that has received the greatest research attention and might be expected to carry the greatest implications for change and disruption, the quantitative evidence itself points to the importance of issues concerned with the preceding relationship between the parent and child, interactions between the gender of both child and parent, social class and material circumstances, continuing family-based relationships and wider social supports.

One of the key features of the empirical work discussed in this chapter is that much of it is strongly oriented to practical outcomes, in relation to therapeutic/medical interventions with individual bereaved children, or in relation to social policy issues. As discussed in Chapter 2, there may be a need for theoretical as well as empirical advances that enable us to see the links between the various contexts and issues surrounding the apparently individual and 'private' experience of bereavement. In the context of children's adjustments to the life changes experienced after divorce or separation, Amato (1993: 35) concludes his review of 180 relevant studies with the suggestion that the intricacies of the evidence points to the need for a *complex model* that considers a variety of resources that may enhance the lives of children, and a variety of stressors that may undermine their well-being, as well as the interaction between these in the lives of individual children: 'The total configuration of resources and stressors, rather than the presence or absence of a particular factor, needs to be considered'.

Writing about the long-term consequences of early adverse family experiences more broadly, Schoon and Parsons (2002) discuss the evidence concerning factors that may 'protect' children and promote their resilience and competence in the face of adversities. They suggest that such factors can be categorized in terms of: characteristics of the children themselves; features of their families; and aspects of their wider social contexts. Certainly the evidence available from the literature on bereavement and young people, concerning the complex ways in which such bereavements may be experienced, suggests that attention needs to be paid to features of all three of these categories (Lutzke *et al.* 1997; Sandler *et al.* 1997). This approach also resonates with that of Thompson's PCS approach (2002) to understanding individual loss and grief, which offers a framework for analysis at various levels: the personal, cultural and structural.

As well as working at different levels, such theoretical models also need to be able to consider processes over time. In the context of bereavement experiences specifically, Clark *et al.* (1994: 129) discuss the *shock/aftershock model*, in which death is understood to trigger a series of changes giving rise to more changes, in ever-expanding circles, 'so that the remainder of the young person's life resounds with the echoes of the parent's death'. The *cascade model* also offers a more complex approach, in which the features of a child's life may be understood in terms of a series of pinball buffers, the pattern and significance of which in future may be altered by the parental death itself, or by secondary effects. In relation to anticipated deaths, Christ (2000: 39) offers the *bereavement outcome model*, which incorporates the illness stage, the child's developmental age group and 'structural dynamic interactive experiences', which include:

> the various pre-existing, death-related and unrelated dynamic (stressful and stress-reducing) interactions that take place between the children, their family, and the larger ecological system they live in, the quality of the grief experience, and the pre-existing attributes in the child and parent that may account for better or more compromised outcomes.

This is in line with Wadsworth's discussion (1991: 140–1) based on the lives of the 1946 cohort by age 36, when he suggests that high scores on emotional distress are likely to be the result of:

> a series or chain of problems . . . [in which] one precipitated another, and . . . social and family circumstances and self-esteem were not strong enough to support the individual at such times . . . Thus, adult vulnerability to emotional difficulties may be the current end point of many earlier experiences of problems, some a matter of bad luck,

some a question of poor self-regard, and others a problem of poor social support; the many interrelationships found between these factors add to the likelihood of strong links perpetuating the chain over many years.

More recently, Amato (2000) offers a model for seeking to understand these complex processes over time, which he calls the *divorce-stress-adjustment perspective*, which could, perhaps, also be usefully applied to research on bereavement. The model sees the original disruption as a process, associated with mediators (stressors) and moderators (protective factors), leading to varied aspects of 'adjustment'.

Schoon and Parsons' (2002: 268) analysis of longitudinal cohort data (the British NCDS and BCS70 data sets, of children born in 1958 and 1970 respectively) points to the need for future research to 'identify specific rather than general protective factors that provide protection against specific risks for young people in specific life contexts'. Their study also found, however, that these protective factors could operate differently for different cohorts of children, and could also vary in their dynamics according to how advantaged the general family context was:

> While in NCDS socially disadvantaged children are negatively afflicted by the experience of long-term separation from the mother and the experience of frequent family moves, socially advantaged children are only slightly influenced by the experience of long-term separation from the mother. In BCS70 life events indicating family instability do not significantly influence the formation of individual competences among socially advantaged children. For socially disadvantaged children in BCS70, however, the experience of being placed in local authority care shows a most devastating negative influence on the formation of individual competences.
>
> (2002: 270)

This discussion points to the need for sophisticated statistical analyses framed by more complex theoretical models that can incorporate attention to structural and cultural issues as well as psychosocial factors, as these occur in interactive processes over time. In the absence of such studies, much of the most contentious debate about 'risk' in relation to young people and bereavement centres on the weight we should place on different aspects of the existing evidence, and the implications this may have for how we respond. We will turn next, in Chapter 5, to a more direct consideration of the social and institutional contexts in which such interventions may be situated.

5 The social contexts of bereavement experiences and interventions

Julie Jessop and Jane Ribbens McCarthy

Introduction

The death of a family member or significant other, while often centred on and in family relationships, has also to be dealt with in a variety of social contexts and institutional settings. Bereavement can be a deeply personal experience and may, indeed, be constructed this way particularly in contemporary western societies (see Chapter 2). Nevertheless, it has to be 'lived', for the most part, within public domains and relationships. The way in which bereavement occurs across the public/private divide, while highlighting the blurred boundaries of such distinctions,[1] also works to illustrate the ways in which emotions have to be 'managed' in varying contexts, and how this can lead to a sense of isolation and individualized pain.

This goes to the 'heart' of issues of emotional control regarding the civilizing process discussed in Chapter 2 – if emotions of grief are too disruptive, how is the individual to 'manage' these in different contexts? Adults may see such emotional disruptions as a reason to avoid some contexts altogether until emotions can be brought under control. In this respect, one important aspect of what is seen as being able to 'cope' or 'function' after a bereavement, is precisely focused on this issue of whether or not it is possible to participate in more 'public' social settings without 'breaking down', in terms of crying or other sorts of 'embarrassing' behaviour (Goffman 1956). It may then be seen as necessary to find 'special' social contexts for dealing with such grief emotions, whether in terms of individual counselling, groups set up specifically for bereaved individuals, behind the closed door of a bedroom, or alone at a cemetery.

In earlier chapters we discussed some of the ways in which bereavement experiences may be mediated by ongoing family-based relationships (Chapter

---

[1] See Ribbens McCarthy and Edwards (2002) for a discussion of some of the ways in which emotion management may be associated with these distinctions.

4), and referred to work that takes a family systemic approach (Chapter 2). Writing in this tradition, Sutcliffe *et al.* point out that 'the interaction of the bereaved with others becomes reactive not just to the event, or to each other, but to the internalised cultural injunctions of "doing it right" ' (1998: ix). The complex effects of loss and shifting relationships, however, do not just impact on (extended) family networks but also on the wider social and institutional affiliations within which young people live their lives. Indeed, it has been suggested that such issues constitute the real crux of bereavement experiences, with bereavement identified in terms of a 'social network crisis' (Vachon and Stylianos 1988 quoted by Hogan and DeSantis 1994: 133). In similar vein, Pietila argues that 'talking about bereavement – in research occasions or otherwise – is [an] utterly social action in which people use culturally and historically specific resources that construct moral orders' (2002: 401).

The social position of 'young people' sees such considerations of moral order and emotional management as significantly heightened during the teenage years. At this point in the life course, part of the social processes in which young people are generally expected to engage is a 'transition' in terms of taking increasing responsibility for the management of their own emotions (see Chapter 2); and part of 'adult' anxieties about teenagers is precisely that they may not be found to be reliable in this respect.

Children and young people may also have little control with regard to whether or not they withdraw or continue to participate in public social settings, particularly in relation to educational institutions. Walter (1999) (and others) highlight the ways in which university students may have to deal with specific issues due to living in two social environments, home and university. While the home may be the site and experience of the bereavement, this may contrast with how they manage their experience at university, where there may be less association with the loss, but the person may not be significant or even known within these other networks.

Other issues may arise for school students about how they deal with the different settings of home and school on a daily basis, though children themselves may hold variable views about whether or how they want these two worlds to connect (see e.g. Edwards and Alldred 2000; Alldred *et al.* 2002). There may be some similar tensions for adults in dealing with emotions of grief in the workplace (see Eyetsemitan 1998).

There are, then, particular issues about how far schools should deal with bereavement issues themselves, or rely on more specialist services in this area. In this chapter some of the issues are writ large in this regard, about how far bereavement can most usefully be understood by reference to its links and continuities with other issues in the lives of children and young people (e.g. as another form of loss or disruption), or by reference to a difference that requires specialist knowledge and interventions from bereavement organizations for children and young people. As Small and Hockey (2001) observe, recent years have seen a proliferation of specialist organizations and related expert discourses and interventions in relation to bereavement issues generally. The discussion of these issues leads on to questions about how far bereavement is a matter of helping specific individual young people who have experienced particularly difficult bereavements, or of understanding death and bereavement as a widespread, 'normal' part of 'growing up' which all children and young people need some help to deal with. Social support issues, however, also raise the possibilities of seeking ways to enable young people generally, whether bereaved or not, to support each other in facing difficult times in life.

This chapter starts by considering research evidence about the implications of bereavement for young people's social relationships beyond the immediate household, as well as ways in which such relationships can mediate or exacerbate some of the impact of bereavement and feelings of loneliness. We move on to consider death and bereavement in the context of educational settings during the teenage years and the potential role of schools in addressing these issues, both in the form of death and/or loss education, and dealing with individual experiences of bereavement. The efficacy of emotional management and literacy is then considered before turning to look at the interventions offered by specialist bereavement organizations. We then assess the overall value of talk and counselling and the role of peers and peer support groups, whether in schools or elsewhere. Finally, we look at the evaluation, or lack thereof, of bereavement interventions and the implications current research carries for both policy and practice. Of course, young people's actual experiences of varying social contacts and contexts are relevant to individual bereavements and, in practice, it may be police or neighbours (Harrison 2001; Leeds Animation Workshop 2002), for example, who are found to be helpful while the educational setting and teachers may be seen as less helpful or relevant.

Loneliness and informal social relationships after bereavement

Popular conceptions of teenagers suggest that friends may become more important than families in the lives of young people. While this may underestimate the continuing significance of family relationships (Gillies *et al.* 2001), bereavement research does point to the key part played by peers, and Walter (1999: 75) suggests in more general terms that 'There is evidence that bereaved persons who are socially isolated are likely to find life particularly hard'. Among young people specifically, research has shown that the presence of close friends can be experienced as extremely supportive, and this is the category most often pointed to as being helpful (Gray 1989; Hogan and

DeSantis 1994; Holland 2001; Rask *et al.* 2002). Furthermore, close supportive relationships with peers may not be seen to carry the potential disadvantages of power differences, control or mutual protection that may be entailed in relationships with parents (as discussed in Chapters 3 and 4, and see Gillies *et al.* 2001).

Some research into the experiences of young people and bereavement has thus paid attention to the implications of, and for, relationships with peers and others beyond the immediate family household. And some studies have pointed to the likelihood of early bereavement having implications (possibly long-term) for social relationships, although this has not received very extensive or systematic attention. The difficulties apparent in wider aspects of contemporary western cultures in dealing with issues of death and bereavement may well thus be felt at the level of individual psychosocial processes associated with a sense of difference and lack of connection.

Issues of social relationships also feature prominently in more qualitative and autobiographical accounts of bereavement (see Chapter 3), and carry implications for how the support needs of these bereaved young people might be met. As an issue, loneliness may interrelate with factors concerning the availability of social support, which may have the potential to mediate some of the negative effects of early bereavement (discussed further below). As various writers point out (e.g. Monroe 1995; Wilby 1995), peers too may need help themselves in knowing how to cope.

Ross Gray (1987) studied 50 young people aged 12–19 whose parent had died during adolescence, and found an association between low social support and high depression scores. There were also lower depression scores among those with religious or spiritual beliefs. Goodman (1986) (discussed by Balk 1995) found that bereaved adolescents who were not in psychiatric treatment found support from the other parent, their peers and other individuals whose parent had died. Balmer (reported in Fleming and Balmer 1996) found that friends were regarded as helpful by some sibling bereaved interviewees, especially if they were friends of the dead sibling. And Schachter (1992), researching 53 young people aged 14–19 who had experienced the death of a peer, found that support from their friends was the most frequently cited source of help.

However, close supportive relationships with a few friends may occur alongside peer relationships that may be experienced negatively, for example in terms of name-calling, bullying etc., and many children and adolescents find that their relationships suffer as their peers have difficulty in understanding what is happening or knowing what to do or say, with potential implications for a sense of isolation (Tyson-Rawson 1996; Worden 1996; Servaty and Hayslip 2001). Calls to ChildLine (the UK anonymous phone helpline available to all children and young people) about bereavement highlight the fact that not only do many children not get the support that they need from their families, but that peers can in fact be extremely hurtful and unsympathetic in the face of loss. 'They laugh at me and call me mumless'; 'My cousin hung himself and they keep telling me they can see things dangling from the trees' (callers to ChildLine, quoted in Cross 2002: 13–14).

In Davies's study of sibling bereavement, loneliness was reported to be a regular problem around the time of death, and this persisted into adulthood: 'siblings respond to the death of a brother or sister with a range of behaviours, most notably they turn inward and become sad and lonely, and with time, they may become socially withdrawn' (1991: 129). Dent *et al.* (1996) similarly found widespread reports of social withdrawal as a response to sibling bereavement. And some researchers (e.g. Murphy 1986 discussed by Balk 1991b) suggest that the greatest sense of loneliness among young people bereaved of a parent may be felt by those who report fewer grief responses.

Tyson-Rawson (1996) points out that studies of bereaved college students generally find that they have difficulties in talking to other students about their bereavement. All the college women in her own study reported difficulties in talking about their experience of paternal death with peers, and might consequently select friends who seemed able to take the death seriously. None felt they could share their bereavement with all their peers: 'Friendships were conducted within an environment that many of the women felt was, at least, unsympathetic and, at worst, hostile. For some adolescents the behaviour of peers tended to make them feel, in the words of one woman, "like a freak"' (1996: 170).

Similarly, Servaty and Hayslip (2001: 331) found that parental death was especially related to feelings and perceptions of being different among adolescents:

> ... findings suggest that parental death is unique in that it disturbs perceptions of interpersonal relationships, a fact which may result in isolation and rob adolescents of needed support at a time when relationships with others (e.g., peers, parents, teachers) are critical to adjustment, well-being, and identity development.

In their general, community-based study of childhood bereavement in Boston, USA (discussed earlier in Chapter 4), Silverman and Worden (1992) found that children who were showing higher levels of affective distress were more likely to experience unsatisfactory peer relationships (discussed by Dowdney 2000). Furthermore, some parentally bereaved children and young people in their study expressed a sense of stigma and being teased (Worden 1996). At one year after the bereavement, a third of children said they felt different, especially older adolescent girls. Nearly half of the children reported a lack of understanding from other children, while children who had been able to talk to their peers had higher levels of self-esteem and self-efficacy.

Social problems and changes in self-perception surfaced by the second anniversary of the death, especially if it was the mother who died, and these problems were more common than in the control group.[2]

In considering relationships beyond the immediate family, other adults may also constitute an important potential resource. Research on divorce points to the crucial part that can be played by strong relationships with another adult or friend (Amato 1993). And Hetherington (2003: 224, 249), in connection with divorce and separation, reports that:

> Almost all of the children who went on to be extremely competent or even good enough had a caring, involved adult in their lives – usually a parent, but sometimes a grandparent, stepparent, teacher or neighbour. However, as the children grew older their relationships with peers and in school also began to influence adjustment ... [a] supportive relationship with a single friend may help to buffer children from the deleterious effects of both peer rejection and marital disruption.

As can be seen, wider adult relationships can thus constitute an important potential source of support. There is, however, very little empirical research concerning the implications of bereavement for a young person's relationships with wider kin (Hogan and DeSantis 1994), and anecdotal evidence suggests that there may be high levels of conflict between a bereaved parent and their in-laws, that might well reduce the availability of these kin as a support for the bereaved child.

Overall, then, there is important evidence that isolation may be a pervasive experience among bereaved young people (as we saw with both Brian and Neville in Chapter 3). Worden, nevertheless, suggests that *not* talking about the deceased 'does not necessarily lead to more emotional and behavioural difficulties' (1996: 53). And a quarter of children in his study, mostly adolescents, were urged by others to show *more* feeling. Adolescents had more difficulty than younger children in talking about their feelings, and this coincides with general issues about appropriate forms of counselling or support specifically for young people (discussed further below).

A number of writers, however, suggest that many young people are not able to talk to anyone at all about their experiences. Murphy (1986) reported that loneliness was a major feature for some bereaved young people aged 18–25 who had been bereaved of a parent between the ages of 3 and 16, whose

---

[2] See also Meltzer *et al.* (2000) who found that the effects of stigma and embarrassment surrounding children's mental disorders (which were in turn significantly associated with some forms of bereavement) could disrupt wider social relationship.

self-esteem was low, and who had low levels of participation in the mourning rituals of their families. In her small-scale study of a school-based sample of bereaved young people, Brown (2002) found that 57 per cent had not talked to anyone about their feelings, the main reasons being fear of upsetting other family members, not knowing where to go for help (this was in a locality where there were well-organized services available, linked to the school), and finding it too difficult or upsetting to talk. In Rosen's study (1984) of young people bereaved of a peer, 76 per cent 'had been unable to share their feelings with *anyone* at the time of the loss and for a long time after' (cited by Ringler and Hayden 2000: 210) – contrasting with the strong support that Maeve found among her friends after the death of their close peers (Chapter 3). In his retrospective study of 70 volunteer interviewees who had been bereaved of a parent during childhood, Holland (2001) found that isolation was a prominent theme, with 56 per cent saying that they had talked to no one about their feelings and experiences. When asked to complete an isolation scale of 0–10, in which 0 indicated the most isolated, almost half of this sample gave a score of 0, and the average score was 2. Isolation has also been identified as a major issue among young people who contact the Cruse internet site for young people (Salter and Stubbs 2004), discussed further below.

The potential role for schools in addressing death and bereavement

Research concerning the significance of peers and other relationships beyond the immediate family points to the importance of schools as a major social context for the bereavement experiences of young people. This, in turn, highlights issues of continuities and discontinuities around the bereavement experiences of young people. In what respects should bereavement be regarded as a majority experience, requiring general provisions for the education of all young people, and in what respects do some bereavements constitute a minority experience, that may require more specialized interventions (of various kinds) than schools can provide?

Here we look specifically at the educational environment as a site within which children and young people spend a large proportion of their time, and in which they have to confront and manage the issues of death and bereavement, both as a means of understanding life, and from having to deal with personal bereavement in the school situation. While there is a growing awareness of the role schools play in teaching children about death – and loss more generally – and also in helping pupils who have experienced bereavement, there are continuing debates about the best way to approach bereavement: whether death should be 'taught' (how and at what age), or how it should be dealt with when it arises.

Because school is where children spend a large proportion of their time, many see it as the obvious setting for both general information to be given, and for intervention to take place, whether we are considering general issues of emotions and mental health (Baring 1999), or bereavement issues more specifically (Schachter 1992; Holland 1993; Gisborne 1995; Wilby 1995; Sheras 2000; Rowling 2003; Wass 2004). Alongside this is a body of research which highlights the impact bereavement can have in schools with respect to disruptive behaviour and loss of concentration, leading to falling grades etc. (Smith and Pennells 1995; Holland 2001; and see discussion in Chapter 4), alongside the wider effects on the school as a whole.

Roeser *et al.* (2001), discussing evidence from the USA and Holland, believe that all youth problems need to be set within a broader framework which includes experiences in various social spheres, including the school, and that the school is a 'normative context of development', affecting social-emotional as well as academic outcomes. Similar arguments are made by some writers in the UK context (e.g. O'Hara 1994; Reid 2002). So far, however, there has been little cross-fertilization of ideas between psychologists interested in clinical issues and educationalists whose main interest is in academic functioning. But, with a growing emphasis being placed on 'mental health promotion strategies' that address both learning and social-emotional concerns, more integrative school-based interventions and practices are being developed. The role of school psychologists is pivotal to this change as a means of looking at ways to 'cultivate the positive' and promote well-being, rather than focus on specific negative behaviour/attitudes.

This review highlights the growing number of initiatives that are being created to help schools deal with both personal bereavements and whole-school crises (e.g. Stokes 2004). However it also shows the lack of any clear guidelines and the resulting randomness of provision (see Rolls and Payne's 2003 review of UK childhood bereavement services, discussed further below). Another disturbing lack is in recognizing that the theoretical emphasis in 'dealing' with bereavement (whether in schools or specialist bereavement organizations) is increasingly embedded, both overtly and covertly, within the contemporary therapeutic framework which places a premium on teaching children to 'express' and '*manage*' their emotions (discussed below). While there is no doubt that this strategy may well help some children and young people to deal with their loss and bereavement, there is also the possibility that for others the failure to 'manage' their emotions according to the culturally prescribed criteria will be further evidence that they are not 'doing it right'.

The academic literature on the role of schools in helping children understand death tends to be split between the issues of general death and loss education, whether being taught as a separate subject or incorporated more generally into other curriculum subjects, and the role of the school in helping individual bereaved children and being able to deal with crisis situations in which the whole school is affected.

Death and bereavement as part of the National Curriculum

Arguments for the inclusion of death education as part of the National Curriculum[3] are based on the view that children have much greater awareness and experience of bereavement and loss than adults tend to perceive (Bowie 2000, and see prevalence statistics discussed in Chapter 1). In the UK, those advocating for death to become part of the National Curriculum believe that in teaching death as part of a natural life-cycle approach, not only would a lot of misinformation and myth be dispelled but, when bereavement does occur, children would be better able to understand and deal with it, whether it was a personal experience or something that was happening to a classmate. Some writers suggest that teaching about death should occur within a broader framework of educating children about issues of 'loss' more generally (discussed by Holland 2001). Understanding and dealing with everyday issues of 'loss', it is argued, could help children and young people improve their abilities to cope with larger losses, and also improve communication with teachers.

Although young people have only recently been consulted in bereavement research, there is growing support from children for the inclusion of death education in the general curriculum. Jackson and Colwell (2001), in a small-scale survey of 14 and 15-year-olds, found that most thought that death should be taught in schools, beginning with primary, and be across the curriculum as part of the life cycle rather than as a specialist subject. Kenny (1998), as part of a qualitative study on young people's attitude to death, found that most 18–23-year-olds that she interviewed believed that death education should be taught in both primary and secondary schools as part of the natural life cycle. However, she highlights that the way in which it is taught is important, and cites instances in the USA where the children, as part of death education in schools, have been asked to make their own wills and design their own coffins; issues that potentially add more controversy to an already difficult subject.

In the UK, Higgins (1999) points out that the 1988 Education Reform Act states that the general principles of the school curriculum are to:

---

[3] 'Death education' is the term most frequently found in the literature which discusses the desirability of including such topics in the school curriculum. While this phrase is certainly succinct and to the point, it does perhaps, in itself, evoke some difficult and negative responses. Alternative terms might, perhaps, be desirable if these issues are to be successfully incorporated into the general school curriculum.

- promote the spiritual, moral, cultural, mental and physical development of pupils at school and of society; and
- prepare such pupils for the opportunities, responsibilities and experiences of adult life.

As such she argues that death should be taught even in primary schools as part of the wider spiritual question of 'whether life has a purpose'. Such themes would certainly resonate with the sorts of existential and religious issues raised by the bereavement experiences of Shirleen and Khattab in Chapter 3.

Wilby, based on her work as a school counsellor in the UK, believes that open discussions would lead to more awareness/ability to cope and stresses that 'The more overt the discussion about death and bereavement, the less fear and mystique which surrounds it' (1995: 240). Mallon, writing from the perspective of a school counsellor in the USA, points out how the reactions of peers to a classmate's bereavement can vary from avoidance to overt forms of discrimination and name-calling. She suggests that these issues can be particularly difficult for boys, who may hide their painful emotions, and their vulnerability, rather than risk being teased or made fun of. It is for this reason that she advocates the teaching of death and bereavement in schools: 'Bereavement and grief may be difficult aspects of the curriculum but they are part of life and schools not only have an important role in responding to loss, they have a crucial role in educating children about it' (1998: 148).

The 'mental health promotion' framework advocated by Rowling is an approach that is more popular in Australia, where death and bereavement studies are a more integral part of the curriculum. Rowling (2003) argues that the public/private distinction between a child's home/school life is a false dichotomy, and that death is not a private issue in the sense that children have to deal with the aftermath within the school environment. (Although see Edwards and Alldred 2000 and Alldred *et al.* 2002 for children's own views about appropriate boundaries between home and school.) Rowling also believes that, because the majority of media portrayals of death are based around trauma and tragedy, 'Schools have a role to play in challenging the negative view portrayed in the media, that loss never has positive outcomes ... A comprehensive approach to loss and grief can develop important life skills in young people and can strengthen school communities' (2003: 1).

In a similar vein, Wass argues for the inclusion of death education in the USA, positing the view that there is a need to normalize 'ordinary' death in order to counteract 'the overwhelming presence of violent death in the entertainment media' (2004: 301). Such approaches are in line with more general discussions of the use of positive youth developmental frameworks in promoting preventive health strategies (Baring 1999). Within such models, death education could be seen as a developmental asset that could be nurtured in all children (Small and Memmo 2004).

The participation of the school in promoting the 'normality' of death is also raised by Stevenson, who argues that it is the school's role to educate 'the "whole child", not some type of disembodied intellect' (2000: 205). Stevenson has designed and taught a high-school death education course in the USA for 25 years, and his views are based on working with young people and adolescents throughout that time. He argues that the belief that children need 'protecting' from death is a misnomer, given that all children experience some form of loss, and that preparing/talking about the subject helps deal with such issues when they arise. The emphasis on 'normalizing' death and bereavement is also evident in research which seeks to promote death being taught across all areas of the curriculum, for example as part of English, science and even maths (Kenny 1998; Job and Frances 2004). Such an approach is in line with the recommendations of the Baring Report in the UK (Baring 1999), which suggested that personal, social and health education (PSHE) should include learning programmes on mental health issues which should be incorporated throughout the curriculum.

It has been argued that one of the main problems with teaching death in schools is the reluctance on the part of staff to take on this role. Many teachers surveyed by Rowling (2003) felt that they were ill-equipped to deal with the subject, or that it was an 'inappropriate' topic to teach. Katz (2001) conducted semi-structured interviews on these issues with teachers and other professionals working in schools over a five-year period. Katz cites Leaman (1995) who suggests that teachers' reluctance to be involved in such issues reflects a particularly English middle-class emotional reserve. Katz concluded: 'the consensus of opinion from those interviewed in my study was that most teachers in the United Kingdom have insufficient preparation to deal with bereaved children and no specific remit to raise these issues' (2001: 149). These findings are echoed by Papadatou *et al.* (2002) who conducted a national survey of teachers in Greece, by Carson *et al.* (1995) who surveyed schools in the USA, and by Leckley (1991) in Northern Ireland (discussed by Holland 2001). Holland argues, however, that many teachers could be helped to undertake work in these areas with training and support, although he found that only 50 per cent of teachers in his UK survey had received any relevant training (Rowling and Holland 2000).

Nevertheless, there is provision for death and loss to be incorporated in areas of the UK National Curriculum. PSHE/citizenship became part of the National Curriculum requirement in English schools in August 2002. It is based on the 'planned provision for emotional and social development' of children (National Children's Bureau 2003), which Job and Francis argue, 'would necessarily include discussion of the life and death continuum' (2004: 8). Its three key elements are for:

- acquisition of accessible, relevant and age-appropriate information;
- clarification and development of attitudes and values that support self-esteem and are positive to health and well-being;
- development of personal and social skills to enable emotional development and interaction with others, as well as making positive health choices and actively participating in society.

In the factsheet on PSHE/citizenship, produced by the National Children's Bureau, (2003), which sets out 'best practice' for schools, the opening paragraph states:

> Children and young people need support in developing emotionally and socially so that they are able to use their thoughts and feelings to guide their behaviour positively and develop personal awareness, emotional resilience and social skills. This will enable them to enjoy and manage their lives now and in the future, be effective learners and active citizens.

This document outlines the significance of a 'whole-school ethos' to promote citizenship, and creative approaches to integrate it into various parts of the curriculum. There is an emphasis on peer education, mediation, support and befriending, but no direct mention of bereavement.

Curriculum 2000, the national PSHE guidelines produced by the government (see www.aas.duke.edu/admin/curriculum2000/report.html), is a 26-page document detailing what should be taught as part of PSHE. The only mention of bereavement comes under Section 3, 'Developing good relationships and respecting the differences between people', where it is stated that one of the things that children should be taught is 'the impact of separation, divorce and bereavement on families and how to adapt to changing circumstances'. Various local education authorities, however, do produce their own information and guidance, for example, the Hertfordshire Grid for Learning, 'Bereavement Loss and Separation', which sets out different ways in which such issues can be integrated into the curriculum (www.thegrid.org.uk/learning/pshe/bereavement). There is also a variety of other curriculum materials for use in this area (e.g. Machin 1993; Ward 1996), and for dealing with death and sudden loss in schools (www.teachernet.gov.uk; www.kented.org.uk/eps-web/teacher_death_and_loss.html). Most recently, the National Children's Bureau, in conjunction with the Childhood Bereavement Network, has provided an extensive discussion and guidelines in relation to bereavement issues in school (Job and Frances 2004).

In some locations, specialist back-up and resources may be available to schools via local hospices and bereavement services (Rolls and Payne 2003). Winston's Wish provides guidelines for schools for responding to a school-related death (Gisborne 1995; Stokes 2004; www.winstonswish.org.uk). Support for more general 'loss' education is provided to schools by Seasons for Growth, an organization which aims to enable pupils to develop knowledge and skills to understand and cope with loss and grief, using facilitated peer support groups (www.goodgrief.org.au/about/what.html).

In the UK, the House of Commons Select Committee on Health (2004), and the government response to this report (Department of Health, 2004), specifically supports the inclusion of death and bereavement as topics within PSHE, along with attendant training for teachers involved in this area, as a way of starting to break down the taboo nature of the subject of death. The inclusion of death and bereavement in the general curriculum is not compulsory however and many schools have tended not to address it because of the difficulties surrounding the subject (Rowling and Holland 2000; Holland 2001). What provision there is, has tended to be random (Rolls and Payne 2003), although provisions and policies in other countries may show a marked difference from this UK picture (Rowling and Holland 2000). How far death and bereavement will in practice be included within teacher training and PSHE remains to be determined.

School-based interventions for bereaved individuals

Although schools have always had to deal with bereavement, this has generally been on an ad hoc basis with no clear understanding of the effects of bereavement on children, and based on individual teachers' attitudes and experiences rather than on any formal training (Eiser *et al.* 1995; Holland 2001). Many schools lack any formal policy of how to respond to a pupil who has suffered a major bereavement (Bullivant 1998; Lowton and Higginson 2002). Over the last decade, however, the role of the school in helping children and young people deal with grief and bereavement has become a topic of debate and controversy (Kenny 1998; Katz 2001). Indeed, Gisborne suggests: 'It could even be argued that a grieving child could fall within the category of having "special educational needs"' (1995: 41).

In line with some of the theories of death and dying (discussed in Chapter 2), Holland and Ludford (1995) argue that to a large extent in western society death has become 'professionalized', and that because most deaths occur in hospital, or the body is quickly removed, children have little natural contact with it and no supportive social mourning practices/rituals, which has led to it becoming a 'taboo' subject. As such, when death occurs, children have little preparation for dealing with it, and it can be frightening and embarrassing for the peer group of the bereaved child (Monroe 1995; Reid 2002) (discussed earlier).

Based on a survey of Humberside schools, Holland (1993) estimates that at any given time up to 70 per cent of schools are dealing with a recently bereaved child (with the death occurring within the last two years), and that, with a growing awareness of both psychological and behavioural problems that can accompany bereavement, teachers themselves need help to under- stand what is happening and to have plans in place to deal with such situa- tions both proactively and reactively. He suggests (2001) that each school should designate particular staff to engage with policies and practices for bereaved children. Similar suggestions are made by Reid (2002), who suggests that all schools should have a member of staff – such as the special educa- tional needs coordinator – who has received training for emotional support. Stokes (2004) in the UK, and Rubel (2005) in the USA, report on the ways in which school nurses may be enabled to take responsibility in these areas, which is in line with suggestions from the Youth Justice Trust in the UK (2003a) for an enhanced role for school nurses in tackling mental health issues generally in schools.

Kenny (1998), in advocating a more integrated school response to death, stresses that many terminally ill children may want to continue attending school for as long as possible, in which case teachers need to be able to deal with it openly rather than ignore it. This point is also raised by Bor *et al.* (2002) who looked at the experiences of two schools dealing with the death of a student: one involving accidental death, and the other based on the an- ticipated death of a pupil through leukemia. They argue that such (antici- pated) deaths are not always easier to deal with as they can unnerve both pupils and staff, leading to restlessness and inattention, and that teachers need to take a lead in helping the class decide how to deal with it rather than ignoring it.

In-depth interviews conducted by Lowton and Higginson (2003) with staff across 13 different London schools found that only one had a specific bereavement policy. In many cases teachers felt they did not have the ne- cessary experience to deal with a child's bereavement and in these cases the children were referred to specialist bereavement services. Dealing with be- reavement in schools also necessitates the need to be aware of individual family structures (which is not always possible in larger school commu- nities) and of the multi-cultural dimensions of a child's life. The 'secret' nature of bereavement also meant that some teachers only found out about significant deaths some time after the event when setting essays in which children had to talk about important life experiences. Other writers suggest that even teachers who have the relevant skills for dealing with bereavement still require further knowledge and reassurance (Druce and Pentland 2004).

Various resources are generally available for schools to provide guidance and advice about how to help bereaved young people, through the websites of national bereavement organizations, and more general educational sites (such as the Scottish Council for Research in Education). In some locations, specialist back-up and resources may be available to schools via local hospices and bereavement services. Rolls and Payne's (2003) UK survey of childhood bereavement organizations found that 66 per cent of these groups were offering services to schools. One of the largest and longest established of these, Winston's Wish, operates in up to 300 schools and provides a 'grief support programme for children', as well as guidelines for schools in how to respond to a school-related death. (Further details of their work can be found in Stokes 2004 and at www.winstonswish.org.uk.) Holland suggests the caveat that: 'The involvement of outside agencies, although perhaps necessary in a small minimum of cases, reinforces the message that death is an unusual event which teachers cannot cope with' (2001: 46). His approach has therefore been to develop a package for training teachers themselves to deal with bereavement issues in schools (Holland 2004). And indeed, some of the work of Winston's Wish has itself been aimed at enabling schools to deal with bereavement issues for themselves (Gisborne 1995). Rainbows is a more broadly focused organization which provides 'training and programmes for children and adolescents who are grieving a death, separation, desertion, divorce or any other painful loss in their family' (www.rainbows.org). These programmes are run through schools, churches and other community services, and are based on peer support groups. (We return to peer support groups below.)

With regard to the views of young people about how schools should deal with individual bereavement, we find a good deal of variability in terms of how, and when, they want schools to be involved (Worden 1996; Holland 2001). While those advocating increased school involvement do so in the belief that interventions will have a therapeutic effect for children, those studies which look at the actual experiences of children involved raise a number of important issues which need to be addressed. Doka (2000) suggests that for some children, especially adolescents, school is not seen as the appropriate place to deal with personal issues. Relationships with teachers and school counsellors are often transitory and fragmented and as such are not seen as relevant. Also, because the aim of many adolescents may be to 'fit in', being singled out for attention, regardless of the intention, can be difficult and lead to further feelings of alienation and loss (Wilby 1995).

Wood and Baulkwill (1995: 167) talked directly to children about their experiences of bereavement and found that how it was handled in the school context was an important issue for them. They quote one child as saying:

> 'A few weeks after my dad died my whole class had to be told about it and my teacher made me tell the class. I would have liked it if the teacher told the class'. Another child was upset because the teacher told the class and he had wanted only a few people to be told. The

overall message is that children's responses vary and they need to be asked how they want it to be handled – none of the children interviewed in this study had been.

The same point is made by Worden (1996) in his two-year study of parentally bereaved children, which found very mixed reactions about school involvement. There was no consensus about the 'right' way to handle it, but individual children needed to be asked how they wanted it done: 42 per cent of teachers told the class about the death, but not all children liked this; a third of children wanted to talk with the teacher and did so; a third wanted to talk to the teachers and the teachers didn't try; and another third (mainly adolescent boys) didn't want to talk but the teachers tried to talk to them. Problems were also reported around the second anniversary of the death, because new teachers were not always aware of the bereavement.

In the UK context, Holland (2004), talking about his previous research with bereaved children, found that children often suffered when returning to school after a bereavement due to mismanagement by teachers. Three quarters of his volunteer sample, of adults bereaved of a parent while a child, said their teachers were not approachable, and more than half felt it would have helped to have someone at school listen to them (Holland 2001). Nevertheless:

> Some children thought *not* being supported actually helped them feel 'normal' ... others thought their teachers had helped them in a variety of ways, such as telling their peers about the death, or acknowledging the loss ... One problem, perceived by many, was the reluctance of teachers and other adults to engage with them, and this seemed to have been constituted as a lack of caring.
>
> (2004: 23)

Reid's (2002) case study of the death of a young girl also highlights the needs of children on returning to the school environment. Both the older siblings of the deceased found that they had little support from their school, and a close friend 'found difficulty expressing his thoughts openly within the school framework', with teachers tending to change the subject when it was broached. This lack of communication was perceived as coming from the teachers' inability to cope with the situation.

One of the difficulties for teachers in both teaching and dealing with bereavement is the duality of roles it can encompass; while the role of the teacher is generally one of control, the issue of death and dying is personal and emotional and can go against previously sustained relationships and roles. Rowling points out that 'One block to the acceptance of grief as a school responsibility is that teachers feel ill equipped' because they're not trained as social workers/psychologists (2003: 8). This again is corroborated by the work of Katz (2001), who also points out that some teachers fear they will do more harm than good by becoming involved, although this seems to be a lesser concern in other national contexts (Rowling and Holland 2000). Katz calls for bereavement issues in particular, and counselling skills in general, to be included in teacher training.

Rowling and Holland (2000) also raise issues of the need for teachers for support *themselves* in dealing with the emotional impact of bereavement experiences. Research by Spall and Jordan (1999) looked at the personal experiences of 11 teachers who had had to deal with bereavement within the school environment. They found that dealing with a bereaved student could leave teachers 'emotionally drained' and with little sense of support or feedback that they were doing the right thing. With respect to the death of a student, teachers often had difficulties in knowing how to talk to a class about it, and also in dealing with their own emotions; only one of the teachers responding had had any relevant training. The issue of teachers' own feelings is highlighted by Rowling (1995) in her work on 'disenfranchised grief'. Here she argues that the professional role of teachers is at odds with what is expected of them when dealing with bereavement, especially when they themselves knew the child involved; the need to be seen to be in control can lead to 'shame' over their own emotions (see also Lowton and Higginson 2002).

Given the ubiquity of bereavement experiences among young people, there may be a strong case for the inclusion of such issues as a core component of teacher training syllabi. Short post-qualifying courses could also be useful for those already trained. Specialists could be available to contribute in specific circumstances – such as sudden and traumatic deaths – taking into account teachers' own feelings about dealing with such issues among their pupils.

Crisis management

Rather different issues arise for schools in relation to traumatic incidents and accidents that occur within the school environment and to members of school communities. While tragic accidents have always happened (e.g. the Aberfan disaster in Wales), large-scale incidents in recent years, both within schools and society generally (such as 9/11, Hillsborough, Dunblane, Columbine High and so on), have heightened concerns about the need for schools to be prepared when a crisis occurs.

Although most schools do not have a pre-planned crisis management policy, either in the UK (Holland 2001; Rowling 2003) or USA (Wrenn 1991; Carson *et al.* 1995), in New South Wales, Australia, each school is legally required to have a 'critical incident' policy (Rowling and Holland 2000). And those schools that have had experience of such a crisis stress the usefulness of a pre-existing plan in dealing with the immediate event and the aftermath (Sorensen 1989; Grant and Schakner 1993; O'Hara *et al.* 1994). The personal experience of a headteacher dealing with a situation in which a pupil was killed during a school trip highlights the necessity of prior planning (Shears 1995). Shears argues that a plan needs to be in place which not only deals with the actual crisis and its effects but also the longer-term consequences for pupils, staff, parents and, in many instances, the wider community, as the school becomes a focal point for the local population. Not only does there need to be a chain of command in which everyone knows what is expected of them, but policies have to be in place to deal with the media and alert other professional agencies which may be needed to help. While schools may not always feel a need to develop their own individual plans, it may be important that they know where and how to access immediate guidelines in the event of actually experiencing such a disaster or critical incident among their own pupils.

In the USA, and in New South Wales, the role of the school psychologist/ counsellor is seen as pivotal in providing crisis guidance and also for organizing support and counselling at the time of the disaster. DeAngelis (2000) argues that in fact the role of the educational psychologist in America is changing from that of an individual assessor to that of a team player working with the whole school/community should tragedy occur. And, although in the UK Holland (1993) found that most schools out of the 75 surveyed would not see this service as particularly relevant or the first point of contact, there is evidence that this may be changing (Holland 2004). The educational psychology service in Salford (O'Hara *et al.* 1994) provides guidelines for schools based on action research following major disasters such as Hillsborough and the *Herald of Free Enterprise*. They emphasize the importance of the input of the educational psychology service in accessing a network of support for both students and staff, to offer both personal and group counselling.

Rickgarn (1996) (USA) talks of the need for 'death response teams' which can be called upon by colleges in times of crisis in order to mitigate both the personal and academic problems that can affect students. Nevertheless, there is continuing debate about whether or not post-disaster trauma is necessarily reduced, or may even be increased, by indiscriminate implementation of counselling services for all those involved.

Whether interventions are geared towards bereaved individuals or towards whole-school crises, one of the main premises they are based on is the need to 'manage' individuals' emotions and it is to this issue that we now turn.

Management of emotions and emotional literacy

As well as pointing to common issues about how to teach other aspects of PSHE, such as sex or drugs education, the potentially disruptive emotions associated with bereavement and grief point to other general debates concerning the relevance and place of emotion management in schools (Weare 2004). Emotional literacy and emotional intelligence have become, over the last ten years, of considerable interest to educationalists and policy-makers, and are based on the view that schools educate the 'whole child' and are not just about transmitting academic knowledge. However, while these terms are often used interchangeably there is a distinction between:

> ... [those] projects that are about instructing young people in how to manage their emotions so as to improve their social behaviour, and those that aim instead to help young people develop levels of emotional understanding that will motivate their desire to learn, enhance their general awareness and stimulate their capacity to engage with questions of values and spirituality.
>
> (Parke 1999: 19)

At present most school projects concerned with emotion and behaviour management, both in the UK and USA, are designed as a way of treating antisocial behavioural problems (Cohen 1999, 2001; Parke 1999; Sharp and Faupel 2002) and, as such, are based on changing the individual rather than looking at the socio-organizational structures which may create such behaviour in the first place. Also, because of the emphasis placed on managing difficult behaviour, Parke argues that such programmes may miss children who do not express emotions and become sullen and withdrawn rather than acting out.

As mentioned above, in the USA it is argued that school psychologists should be at the forefront not only of dealing with crises but also in advocating, developing and implementing programmes dealing with death education, although this may require a high level of communication between practitioners and schools to be successful (Douglas *et al.* 2004). Aspinall (1996: 346) argues that although their role is generally seen as interventionist, there is a need for a more educative approach to help students understand the normality of life and death and develop 'effective coping strategies which will enhance students' ability to communicate and *manage their emotions*' (emphasis added).

In this respect, death education as a spiritual and practical issue may also, arguably, be broadened out to include the more emotional aspects of grief and bereavement. Sharp defines emotional literacy as 'the ability to recognise, understand, handle, and *appropriately express* emotions' (2000: 8, emphasis added; cf. Goleman 1995). He is a strong advocate of its incorporation into the curriculum and all other aspects of schooling, and instrumental in various initiatives run by the Southampton local education authority in the UK (for details see www.nelig.com/PDT/selig_guidelines.pdf).

The US series on social emotional learning (SEL) (Cohen 1999, 2001) is largely based on Goleman's 'emotional intelligence' (1995), and the belief that emotional well-being is a better predictor of life satisfaction than academic performance. Cohen's main contention is that 'Awareness of ourselves and others provides the foundation for social and emotional competencies: a sense of self-worth' (1999: vii). He argues that such awareness comes from the ability to be self-reflective, and his edited series sets out various ways in which children can be taught/encouraged to become more self-reflective in developmentally appropriate stages. However, there is an admission that little research into the efficacy of SEL programmes has so far been carried out, although Newman (2002) suggests that such programmes can enhance children's resilience.

The belief in the effectiveness/desirability of teaching emotional literacy in schools has, indeed, been criticized, especially in the UK where there appears to be a more critical appreciation and a greater recognition of the cultural/historical specificity of these attributes/abilities. (See the work on the sociology of emotions, as well as Foucauldian analyses of increasing discourses of self-surveillance, discussed in Chapter 2.) Burman (2000) questions the way in which the current confessional and therapeutic popular culture of catharsis and self-enlightenment has extended into the educational arena, resulting in a convergence between educational and therapeutic discourses.

The philosophical and ethical concerns associated with the belief that emotional literacy can (and should) be 'taught' are outlined by Carr. He argues that the way in which emotional intelligence is being introduced into the curriculum is via a 'covertly "naturalistic" therapeutic way as though we were all absolutely clear and agreed about what constitutes appropriate and inappropriate, healthy or diseased, ways of handling or expressing affect' (2000: 29). From the perspective of morality he points out that 'people who are poor at controlling their emotions and feelings (who, for example, are easily moved to tears or anger) may be morally preferable to those who are particularly good at controlling their own feelings or intuiting the feelings of others' (p. 31). Furthermore, Carr argues, such 'skills' can lead to emotional cleverness and cunning, to negative as well as positive outcomes.[4] Carr believes that in attempting to solve problems associated with poor schooling outcomes, people have been quick to see emotional learning as a panacea, and that little attention has been paid to 'the ethical and eva-luative complexities in which any talk of emotional intelligence cannot but be implicated' (p. 32).

If emotional literacy is to be pursued in schools it will need to be sensitive to cultural differences (whether related to gender, class, race, disability etc.) with respect to what is considered to be the appropriate expression of emo-tions. It will also need to avoid therapeutic assumptions of the value of talk and emotional expression (discussed below), and to take account of young people's own views of the desirability of keeping personal and private boundaries around their school lives (Edwards and Aldred 2000; Alldred et al. 2002). Given these parameters, it may have a part to play in helping young people consider their own emotions – including grief – and those of their peers.

Specialist bereavement interventions by voluntary organizations in the UK

While schools and teachers may still be exploring how far, and in what ways, they should deal with bereavement issues within the education sector, spe-cialist bereavement organizations in the voluntary sector have been devel-oping their own services for children and young people, both in terms of providing support and advice to schools, and in terms of providing services directly to bereaved individuals outside the school setting (Rolls and Payne 2003). And, while this may arguably have initially happened 'with minimal national debate and no agreed standards or guidelines' (Stokes et al. 1999: 291), May 2001 saw the advent in the UK of the Childhood Bereavement Network, enabling people to work towards increasing support for, and co-ordination of, services. The Network, operating within the auspices of the National Children's Bureau, has guidelines for best practice that cover such issues as safety, practice context, quality and accountability, and equality.

Rolls and Payne's (2003) survey of childhood bereavement services available in the UK points out that the last decade has seen an increase in more formalized bereavement provision, with 35 per cent of the organiza-tions indicating that they had started their service since 1998. The survey

---

[4] Hetherington (2003) provides evidence of the development of these sorts of skills in 'manipulation' by some children of divorced or separated parents, who in many ways appear to have positive outcomes in their adult lives.

found that 86 per cent of services offered interventions to children and young people up to age 18, with only 3.3 per cent specifically targeting 11–18-year-olds, and the remaining organizations restricting their clients to children aged under 14 or even younger. Cruse, the major UK national bereavement organization, has established an interactive website specifically for bereaved young people (Crusenews, summer 2003), with opportunities for participants to exchange messages and to make their experiences and feelings known and available to others. (Available at www.rd4u.org.uk, or via the Cruse website, www.crusebereavementcare.org.uk, then click Youth Involvement Project.) And Winston's Wish has also developed a website aimed at 12 to 18-year-olds (www.winstonswish.org.uk). Such web-based services and email support carry the potential for both advantages and disadvantages compared with face-to-face work (Salter and Stubbs 2004; Stokes 2004).

The availability of childhood bereavement services, however, is predominantly (86 per cent) based on geographical location. Also, of the 91 organizations identified by Rolls and Payne (2003) as providing services for children, 85 per cent were voluntary sector (although funding arrangements often included government money), and 41 of the voluntary sector services were located in hospices. Of bereavement services for children and young people, 75 per cent could be regarded as specialist organizations in the sense that their remit was specifically focused on issues of bereavement and/or care of the dying. The remaining 25 per cent were part of other organizations, such as the NHS, or more general counselling services. There was also a great range in the nature of the services or interventions being offered (e.g. 36 per cent did not offer interventions with children or young people as individuals).

Stokes *et al.* (1999) point out that, in the late 1990s in the UK, although the hospice movement had highlighted, and was increasingly providing for, situations where death had been anticipated, there remained little support for those cases where children were bereaved following sudden death. Rolls and Payne (2003) thus make a clear distinction between 'open access' and 'closed access' services, with regard to the types of death covered (with 71 per cent of services being open in this respect), and whether or not specific referral agents were required (with 71 per cent of services also being open in this regard). Alongside this, Stokes *et al.* suggest that, because of the lack of resources, it is only when a bereaved child is exhibiting signs of disturbed behaviour that referrals are made to statutory services, and a child may have to wait more than six months before being seen.

The situation remains, then, that availability of counselling and other bereavement support services for bereaved young people may be completely absent in some localities, and may be contingent in others. We do not have any evidence about the numbers of bereaved children who have no access to such non-clinical services through these sorts of reasons. Even in those areas where a service is available, it may only be able to offer interventions with a very limited number of children: Rolls found that 35 per cent of organizations saw less than 25 children each year, while, at the other end of the scale, 19 per cent saw over 100 children a year. Services may also be limited in terms of the type of bereavement concerned (e.g. 18 per cent of services working only with children who had lost a sibling). Rolls and Payne (2003) conducted case studies within eight of the identified organizations and found that services continue to be 'very diverse'.

Drawing on the work of Worden, Stokes *et al.* (1999) discuss three possible models for the provision of support services to bereaved children:

1   to provide services to those children who 'display levels of emotional and behavioural problems or psychological distress' (p. 294);
2   to provide services to those children 'identified *at risk* by use of a screening measure' (p. 294);
3   to offer services routinely to all bereaved children and their families (later defined by reference to children bereaved of a parent or sibling).

These authors go on to argue the merits of the third model in the UK context (as does Winton 2002 and see also Stokes 2004). These services, they suggest, should be funded by monies specially raised in local communities, and provided in settings outside statutory mental health services, which may be less stigmatizing (Meltzer *et al.* 2000), although referrals would be made to mental health services as necessary. In the experience of one such locally-based service – St Christopher's Hospice in London – only 10 per cent of children needed more than six sessions. And other writers offer discussion of factors that might indicate a particular need for interventions with certain individuals (e.g. Black 1998; Holliday 2002).

As Rolls points out, however, we have no information about the social processes that may lead to interventions being offered to children and young people, with regard, for example, to such issues as social exclusion. Gersten *et al.* (1991) found that surviving mothers were much more likely to seek help for their paternally bereaved children than were surviving fathers for maternally bereaved children. The paternally bereaved children who were referred for help by their mothers had very high levels of conduct disorder, unlike the parentally bereaved children generally in their community-based sample. A further concern is raised by Stuber *et al.* (2002), however, since they found that, in their study of post 9/11 trauma in Manhattan, it was the level of the parent's stress, rather than the child's, that related to children and young people being referred for counselling.

This points to the potential importance of facilitating young people's own direct access to information, support and services. In the broader context of young people's mental health needs, the Mental Health Foundation (Baring 1999) has pointed to the need for a national strategy for the provision of information, advice and counselling needs, with a recommendation for informal, flexible and easily accessible points of contact for young people seeking help. Holland's retrospective study (2001) of adults bereaved as children found that many of them lacked basic information around the time of the death, and lacked the power to gain such information. As we saw with Neville's case study in Chapter 3, it is clear that family members do 'protect' each other from knowledge of each other's distress. Would Neville have taken up opportunities to talk (outside of the research interviews in which he was involved) if they had been available to him, and what format would have been appropriate? How could he have accessed them? The small UK study by Brown (2002), of bereaved young people in two secondary schools, is important in showing the extent to which young people were unaware of services available to them, even in a locality where service provision was relatively available and well-organized. This suggests the importance of provision of information to young people in ways that are easily accessible to them, as well as the provision of services as such.

Referral processes to bereavement organizations in the first place, either in practice or ideal, are not discussed at all by Stokes *et al.* (1999) in their review and discussion of bereavement services for children and young people in the UK. This issue is, however, the focus of the research by Dowdney *et al.* (1999) located in London, who found that 60 per cent of parents in their study stated their wish for services to be provided for their child/children. This is in line with the findings of Dent *et al.* (1996 cited by Holliday 2002), that two thirds of families where a child had died were not satisfied with the professional support available to the surviving siblings. While Dowdney *et al.* (1999: 356) do not explicate what sort of services were being considered in their study (the implication seems to be that they were concerned with statutory services), they found, disturbingly, that the likelihood of receiving support from services:

> ... was unrelated to probable psychiatric disturbance in children or parents or to parental desire for support ... It was only the child's level of disturbance that significantly influenced parental desire for service support. Yet those most likely to be offered service provision were families in touch with services before the death ... These findings indicate a serious mismatch between service need and provision.

In general terms, young people themselves, as a group, may have little awareness of the range of general services available to them, and find them hard to access when they do try to do so. Studies of those most likely to use general services indicate that it is the more privileged, and those with supportive families, who are likely to access help (Tijuis *et al.* 1990 cited by Griffiths 2003) and to have positive expectations about the possibilities for change.

Dowdney *et al.* suggest that GPs and primary health workers may have a particular role to play in this regard. Supporting this concern, Lloyd-Williams (1999) suggests that one of the problems may be that primary health care workers are not trained in these issues, and fail to link problems presented at the surgery with an earlier bereavement. This resonates with the recommendations of the Baring Inquiry in the UK (Baring 1999), that GPs and psychiatrists both need better training in listening and communication skills in order to be able to help effectively with young people's mental health issues. Black provides some suggestions for how GPs might organize their responses to childhood bereavement in particular, suggesting that: 'Preventive counselling is properly the responsibility of the primary care team, utilising the resources of bereavement counselling services as necessary' (1998: 933).

In the context of sudden deaths, particularly, Smith and Browne (2004) suggest that hospitals may also have an important part to play in ensuring that, where no other support is in place, affected children are identified and referred to a bereavement facilitator. However, surveys by the Department of Health (2001, 2004) show little evidence of hospitals having provisions or policies for responding to bereaved children and young people. A variety of general professionals could also act as sources of information after bereavement, including funeral directors and clergy. These issues of accessing support after bereavement parallel discussions about the provision of help services more broadly to young people (Griffiths 2003).

There are, then, various possible formats in which support for bereaved young people may currently be provided, or could be provided. Underlying some of the uncertainties about how to provide services in relation to bereaved young people are debates about the point at which grief reactions should be classed as 'pathological' and how 'normal' grief should be supported. The issues regarding such boundaries need to be addressed. Following on from some of the discussion in Chapter 4, when we considered the confusion that may be generated by the failure to distinguish clearly enough between bereavement as a risk factor for clinical/pathological depression, and bereavement as occasioning distress, there is a parallel source of confusion in some of the debate regarding interventions. Clinical depression would seem to point to a need for interventions from mental health professionals, whereas distress may point rather to a need for the availability of empathetic supportive help. This raises issues about how far it is helpful to see bereavement and grief as associated with 'normal' or 'pathological' behaviours. These issues are explicitly addressed by Stokes *et al.* (1999) who suggest that there may be different levels of skills and training needed in various contexts for helping bereaved children and young people, but that community-based services should routinely be offered to all bereaved children and their families (see also Stokes 2004). However, issues remain about how such a universal service may be delivered and to whom. These writers are focused on bereavement through death of a parent or sibling, so are omitting those bereaved of a peer. Furthermore, young people at risk of social exclusion may be the ones most likely to be without any access to services (Rolls and Payne 2003), and there may be particular issues about how to fund and provide community services in particularly deprived areas. Yet these areas may be the ones where support is most needed by bereaved children, given that young people in such areas are more likely to experience significant bereavements in their lives (see Chapters 1 and 4), and to be living in localities where others' own resources to provide support have been depleted by a variety of stresses.

However, other debates about the provision of services to bereaved young people extend into further issues concerning the aim and form of interventions, such as controversies surrounding the 'management' of emotions (discussed above), counselling as a useful support service and the value of talk more generally.

How valuable is talk and counselling?

While voluntary organizations have been seeking to develop their services in response to what is seen as an urgent set of unmet needs, there is an ongoing (sometimes fierce) debate about how far counselling can appropriately ease the 'normal' distress of grief and, more specifically, whether talking can help. Furthermore, the usefulness of talk generally may be significantly shaped by factors of class, culture and gender (Seale 1998; Strange 2005). However, such issues are not generally raised in the literature concerning bereavement interventions. Small and Hockey discuss ways in which theories of grief and bereavement (as discussed in Chapter 2) may shift from their basis in (clinically theorized) descriptions of how people may feel or behave after bereavement, into becoming normative expectations about how people should react, and thence into forms of intervention intended to help people to fulfil these. Small and Hockey argue that the guidance offered by various key writers for counselling bereaved people, or even for those who are simply in contact with them, represents a 'hybrid construction' between the 'theoretical substratum' and 'operational practice' (2001: 112).

A sociological analysis of bereavement counselling is offered by Seale (1998) who suggests that psychological interventions, such as bereavement counselling, lead to a 'restructuring of biography' and 'the containment or the "placement" of disorderly experience and behaviour' (p. 196), promoting the restoration of ontological security as well as the development of social cohesion through the reaffirmation of continuing social bonds. He discusses counselling and support groups in terms of 'performative ritual' through which ideas of 'the grief process' are used to define 'normality' and membership of an 'imagined community'. He raises questions regarding the power/status processes involved in these activities, and the possibility that such rituals may be imposed on people. Drawing on the work of Danforth, he suggests that mourning rituals are 'a concrete procedure ... for the maintenance of reality' (p. 202). Routine practices may be a way of creating a negotiated social order that can help prevent insecurities. Drawing on those sociological theories of phenomenology and symbolic interaction which focus on the ways in which social life is created and sustained in daily social interactions, such an analysis can thus point to the significance of talk in everyday interaction, not just in counselling settings, in maintaining and constructing a sense of reality that 'keeps at bay the existential threat posed by human mortality' (Walter 1999: 70). Such a perspective leads Walter to argue that 'the interpersonal processes of integration and regulation [of which talk is one part] can be *as* important as any intra-personal processes' (p. 124). Nevertheless, it is important to recognize that such interpersonal processes need not necessarily be significantly based in talk, as we see in Strange's (2005) description of the largely silent gatherings of concerned friends and neighbours after a bereavement in working-class households in the UK at the turn of the twentieth century.

In less academic terms, the extent to which debates about the value of talk can be a focus of public controversy can be exemplified by the *New Scientist* article, titled 'Counselling can add to post-disaster trauma' (Coghlan 2003). In this article, psychologist Simon Wesley of King's College London is quoted as saying: 'We have an ideology that it's "good to talk", but sometimes that's not so'. However, the article derives from an evaluation study by Wesley of a very specific service, which was a particular form of one-off bereavement counselling offered in the immediate aftermath of a disaster.

Discussing young people's support needs more generally, Hill (1999: 139) suggests that 'the typical young person has little idea of the role of psychiatrists, psychologists or social workers, and for the most part no wish to consult them'. Research practice with adolescents with general mental health difficulties confirms that this age group can be very 'hard to reach', with over 80 per cent of those in need failing to receive appropriate services (Griffiths 2003). Self-referrals are rare, with reliance instead on peers and sometimes family members, particularly mothers.

Harrington and Harrison (1999) question whether bereaved children and young people necessarily either need, or will benefit from, counselling interventions. In their subsequent community-based research, Harrison and Harrington (2001) found that 87 per cent of bereaved adolescents said they 'had never, rarely or only sometimes talked about the deaths of relatives or friends' (p. 163), and 'talking about deaths was associated with higher levels of depressive symptoms'.[5] The vast majority (88.5 per cent) also said they 'never or only rarely needed professional help for the way they were feeling about the deaths they had experienced'. Harrington and Harrison therefore conclude that 'there is little support, then, among adolescents themselves for the widespread development of specialized bereavement counselling services' (p. 164).

This conclusion, however, does seem to go beyond what is warranted by their data, since we cannot know what sorts of professional help young people may have had in mind, or have had experience of, when they said they did not need such help. Young people were not asked directly if they would have liked more opportunities to talk about their feelings. This was also the case with the research by Dowdney *et al.* (1999), who asked parents and teachers about the experiences of children and young people, but did not ask young people themselves about their experiences and views on desirable support. In his work on the therapeutic benefits of narrative work as a form of intervention based on meaning reconstruction theories (discussed in Chapter 2), Neimeyer (2002: 63–4) is concerned to stress that:

> Nothing in what we have said is intended to imply that all bereaved persons undertake an agonizing search for philosophic meaning in their loss, or that professionals should instigate such a search when the bereaved themselves do not do so. Indeed, a minority of even traumatically bereaved persons – about 15 per cent according to the best available data – seem to cope practically, straightforwardly and successfully without such an explicit search.

Brown (2002) also discusses other work about the reluctance of adolescents to seek professional help for emotional problems. She argues that Harrington and Harrison are wrong to equate low levels of counselling for bereaved adolescents with lack of a need for counselling. She presents evidence about bereaved young people not knowing about possible services (though it's not clear they would have used them if they had known about

---

[5] The query does arise, however, whether those who talked a lot might be more willing to describe depressive symptoms, and whether those who are referred for services might be more willing to 'admit' to symptoms. (This is relevant to Downey *et al.*'s (1999) findings too.) It is also an open question whether the most depressed individuals felt the greatest urge to talk, or whether talk itself increased depression.

them), and fear of upsetting other family members, alongside evidence from other studies about parents' difficulties in talking to young people about grief.

In discussing young people's use of services in general, Hill (1999: 135) concludes:

> Many young people are suspicious of professionals who are strangers to them. Children also want to be treated as whole human beings, not simply in relation to one 'problem' or 'disorder' ... Among the implications for professionals are that effective direct work requires the opportunity to establish trust over time. In many circumstances, it may be more productive to work with the people in a child or young person's social network whom they already have confidence in.

Hill suggests that young people may generally have a variety of strategies for dealing with problems such as listening to music or being alone, but for many, talking and listening may be one important outlet. A study specifically of young people bereaved of a peer found that hugs, talk and listening were all felt to be helpful, although often too limited in time (Ringler and Hayden 2000). Young people who have experienced a mental health crisis have also been found to value talk and listening (Leon and Smith 2001 cited by Griffiths 2003).

However, many services for bereaved young people recognize that talk and individual counselling is not always the most appropriate form of intervention for everyone (Silverman 2000). Other approaches are increasingly being offered instead, including play therapy (Webb 2000), ritual (Doka 2000), creative strategies (Fry 2000), or books (Corr 2000b). And some interventions offered may involve only a brief time scale (Monroe and Kraus 2005). As an alternative to individual help, interventions with families may offer an entirely different theoretical and practical approach (Sutcliffe *et al.* 1998; Grollman 2000; McBride and Simms 2001; Kissane and Bloch 2002) – although these are also generally centred on talk.

Talking with peers

Given young people's frequent reluctance to talk to adults, and need to establish trust in the context of unequal power relationships (Hill 1999), and given the significance attached to support from friends discussed earlier, peer group interventions might seem to have much to offer to vulnerable young people (Cowie 1999; Johnson 2002). Peer group support is, therefore, one avenue that may seem attractive as an intervention for a variety of reasons. Facilitated peer group support for young people may be located either in school settings (in which case it is not likely to be focused primarily on bereavement issues, or even family disruption or relationship issues more generally) or in dedicated settings specially created by bereavement organizations as part of the interventions they offer (in which case, they may also create support groups for specific bereavement experiences, such as loss through suicide).

Support groups, both for children and adults, work on the assumption that individuals benefit from 'sharing with "fellow sufferers", that is, a private as well as a public matter' (Pietila 2002: 403). Newman (2002) suggests that peer support groups can enhance children's resilience, while Tedeschi (1996) believes that group work with bereaved young people helps overcome isolation and helps to both 'contain' and 'express' emotions in a supportive setting, linking the proliferation of 'mutual help' groups in the USA with the beginning of Alcoholics Anonymous in the 1930s.

In a similar vein, Sharp and Cowie (1998) highlight the effectiveness of holiday camps for bereaved children and see their success as allowing children to talk to each other: 'it has been found that talking to other bereaved peers is one of the most therapeutic forms of intervention in coming to terms with a death' (1998: 48). However, Pietila (2002) argues that this can lead to those who are seen to fail in demonstrating the 'appropriate' emotions, or ability to talk, being considered cold and indifferent (and see the earlier discussion about emotional literacy).

Silverman (2000), based on her work with bereaved children and adolescents, while acknowledging that 'other people do not always help', believes that schools not only have a duty to teach children about death but that they should also facilitate the formation of group support to help children in similar situations. Currently in the UK, however, peer group support for bereaved young people is almost entirely based in specialist bereavement organizations, with 45 per cent of childhood bereavement services in Rolls's UK survey offering support groups. This compares with the earlier study by Wright *et al.* (1996) of six hospices in the UK, in which it was found that none of these organizations were offering support groups for children at that time. (And see earlier discussion of the work of Winston's Wish and Rainbow in the UK context).

In the UK, the Peer Support Forum was founded by the Mental Health Foundation and ChildLine in 1998, and is currently part of the Children's Development Unit (www.ncb.org.uk/psf/). The aim of the Forum is to encourage schools to facilitate students to offer help and support to fellow students; projects remain under the direction and control of each individual school and can be implemented as listening services or as mentoring and befriending schemes (Cowie and Sharp 1996). The main issues that currently seem to be addressed by such schemes are those of bullying and racism, although some research points to the effectiveness of whole-class groups in

improving peer interactions around various aspects of family change (Douglas
et al. 2004) (and see the work of Jigsaw4u at www.jigsaw4u.org.uk/aboutus/
aboutus.asp). The desirability of extending such schemes to cover more
'personal', family-related topics may be linked with issues of emotional
literacy.

The value of talk, as a major feature of much bereavement intervention
work, leads on to the question of the need for evaluation of all the various
forms of intervention that may be offered.

Evaluating interventions

While there is strong evidence for the effectiveness of early intervention work
in schools for reducing mental health problems among children and young
people (Durlak cited by Baring 1999), the evaluation of different types of
intervention in response to bereavement is a much debated issue. Numerous
publications provide qualitative accounts (often underpinned by strong beliefs) of the positive benefits for children and young people in being involved
in some form of intervention programme after a major bereavement (e.g.
Wolfe and Senta 1995, 2002; Sharp and Cowie 1998). There have also been
numerous quantitative evaluation studies that have sought to assess the effectiveness of such interventions. However, there are serious methodological
problems with the great majority of these studies. These include the ethics of
controlling individuals' access to services for research purposes, the nature of
the outcome being measured, and the enormous range of different sorts of
intervention that may be offered (Schneiderman *et al.* 1994; Stokes *et al.* 1997;
Curtis and Newman 2001; Schut *et al.* 2002).

There is also a question mark over how to measure the effectiveness of an
intervention. Should it be measured on the basis of participants' own views or
by reference to measured outcomes (Stokes *et al.* 1997; Small and Hockey
2001)? Some evidence also suggests that the effectiveness of therapeutic interventions generally varies according to the level of motivation of those
taking part (Garfield 1994 cited by Schut *et al.* 2002). This is in line with the
discussion in Chapter 4 concerning the significance of individual meanings in
mediating the impact of bereavement generally, but again, it increases the
complexity of evaluating interventions. Stokes *et al.* (1997) stress the need for
evaluations that measure outcomes that are appropriate for the aims of the
service, and that consider the implications for families as an interacting
process, rather than just for children as individuals.

Quantitative evaluation studies have generally focused on programmes
offered to *all* children who have been significantly bereaved rather than
programmes that specifically identify bereaved children considered to be at
increased risk. Two relevant reviews (Schneiderman *et al.* 1994; Curtis and

Newman 2001) find the evidence to be too inconclusive to be able to re-commend such interventions. Curtis and Newman therefore recommend against the provision of routine services for bereaved children, although this conclusion seems to be a matter of personal judgement. Meanwhile, Har-rington and Harrison (1999) suggest the possibility of active harm resulting from such interventions, although none of the evaluation studies we con-sidered gave evidence of such harmful effects. Others, however, interpret the evaluation studies more favourably for interventions with children and young people in particular, suggesting that there is more evidence that such children's programmes do help them cope with their loss than there is for adult intervention programmes (Schut et al. 2002; Schut 2005). And a more recent random controlled trial study in the USA of a family bereavement programme for families who were not already receiving interventions and were not showing signs of existing mental health problems (Sandler et al. 2003), found the programme to be effective in improving both family and individual risk and protective factors in the short term, although this was sustained in the longer term only for girls and for those who had higher problem scores at the outset.

Bereavement support groups for children that are based in a medical centre rather than in a school have been assessed as effective by Wolfe and Senta (2002). Their research is based on the Young Person's Grief Support Program (YPGSP) in the USA that has been facilitating bereavement groups for children and adolescents for the last 11 years. In total over 600 children have taken part in the groups and, although Wolfe and Senta recognize that not all young people and their families benefit from such groups, they stress that: 'We strongly believe that bereavement support groups for youngsters facilitate children's healthy adjustment to the death of a parent, sibling, grandparent, relative or friend' (p. 203).

From a psychiatric perspective, group bereavement work in the USA has been assessed as effective in dealing with both children bereaved by suicide (Pfeffer et al. 2002), and with survivors of homicide victims (Salloum et al. 2001). Saltzman et al. (2001) screened young people via schools for experience of any general severe exposure to community violence, then offered sup-portive group programmes and found a reduction in levels of trauma.

In a different, but related context, peer support group interventions, set up specifically to deal with primary-school children whose parents were di-vorcing, were looked at by Wilson et al. They studied both individual and group interventions within the school setting for children. In total 69 chil-dren (aged between 5 and 11) took part and were randomly allocated to either the group or individual intervention. Psychometric measures, together with parent, child and teacher reports, were taken prior to the intervention, dur-ing, and six months following. They found that 'although children who took part in the groups were generally more positive about the support, children in the individual format showed the greatest improvements according to the psychometric measures' (2003: 19). One of the issues raised by this study, however, was that of confidentiality, with some children finding it difficult not to talk to others (including parents) about issues that had been raised in the groups. This sort of study, then, again raises issues about how to measure effectiveness – by reference to the participants' own views or by reference to measured outcomes (Small and Hockey 2001)? It is also likely that such schemes may raise some different issues in relation to young people in secondary schools.

The usefulness of peer support groups, specifically with respect to bullying, has been studied for a number of years by Cowie (1998, 2000) as part of research funded by The Prince's Trust. A report by Cowie *et al.* (2002: 453) looked at how such groups had evolved in 35 secondary schools. They found that generally, although problems existed with respect to the recruitment and retention of boys into these groups, 'There was widespread support for the systems and a strong sense that both teachers and peer supporters were increasingly confident about the value of their service'.

Overall, it is clear that more and better evaluation studies of different forms of bereavement intervention are needed. In addition to the requirement for methodological rigour, these need to cover a range of different sorts of intervention, referral processes and outcome measures, alongside 'an assessment of naturally occurring social support before, during and after the intervention takes place' (Schut *et al.* 2002: 732).

There is also argument to be made for a greater range of methodologies for studying outcomes, including qualitative techniques (Curtis and Newman 2001). And there is scope, too, for broadening out from studies of bereavement interventions to consider what is to be learned from evaluations of other sorts of intervention programmes with young people.

However, given the complexity of the issues to be addressed by rigorously quantitative evaluation studies of the variety of interventions, it may be unrealistic to defer providing such services until there is a quantitative evidence base to underpin them. Peer group interventions generally appear to be well supported by evaluation research, and there is no evidence that interventions with individual bereaved children result in any harm, but some evidence that they can indeed be useful, particularly for some groups of children and young people.

Conclusions

In this chapter we have discussed some of the issues surrounding the bereavement experiences of young people by reference to their peer relationships and other relationships beyond the family. Very little research has been concerned with the latter, and the former question has not been a major focus for outcome research (as discussed in Chapter 4). There is, however, evidence of the importance of peer relationships, both positively and negatively experienced, along with some suggestion of the possibility of loneliness as a (long-term) outcome of significant bereavement for some young people. It is also clear that many bereaved young people do not talk to anyone about their grief, although it is not apparent how many of these would like opportunities to talk, nor to whom.

While there would seem to be some forceful arguments for including 'death (and loss/change) education' in the general school curriculum, it seems likely that teachers generally feel ill-equipped to deal with it, so that its implementation in the UK seems to be rarely undertaken – although we have no research evidence to know for certain on this point. Its general inclusion in the curriculum would seem to have much to recommend it, both as a means of educating young people as individuals, and also as a means of equipping them to offer support to others when needed.

There are ongoing, fierce debates about whether or not help with grief is something that all young people may need, or would benefit from, and, if so, what might be the most appropriate setting for providing such help. There might, in the long run, be a risk of conveying a message to young people that a major crisis, such as a significant bereavement, is difficult to manage without organized support. Interventions thus need to build on young people's existing informal supports wherever possible. Peer support groups, whether in schools or provided by bereavement services, therefore appear to have particular advantages. At the same time, the general privatization and medicalization of death and bereavement may have disabled informal sources of support from being effective, and several studies point to an absence of support or information from more general professionals, such as teachers, clergy and general medical personnel.

It is crucial to distinguish here between policies to make services *available and known* to all who might want them, and policies aimed at *providing* them as a matter of course for all bereaved children. Overall, a range of supports is likely to be needed, given the variety of ways that individual young people cope with difficulties in their lives. Such supports might range, for example, from basic information and acknowledgement concerning the death, to direct interventions. Certainly young people's need for information and clear communication is stressed by many writers (e.g. Rosenheim and Reicher 1985 cited by Black 1998; Holland 2000; Holliday 2002). Support may also need to be available over a much longer time period than is generally the case at present.

A range of mainstream services – including schools, hospitals and GP practices – could provide the framework for routine community-based sources of information, support and referral for bereaved young people. Services need to be made available to young people bereaved in a variety of circumstances, whether the death is of a peer, a close friend, or an unborn child, as well as those bereaved of a family member. For such provision to be possible, such services are likely to need to have both policies in place, and designated individuals who have been appropriately trained to be able to help.

Such interventions need to be better evaluated and coordinated across the range of service providers, including school nurses, educational psychologists, teachers, primary health care workers, mental health professionals, youth workers and voluntary bereavement counselling services. This is in line with the recommendation made by the Mental Health Foundation inquiry for the development of the capacity of mainstream services to recognize and begin to meet the needs of children and families when difficulties arise: 'One of our main conclusions is that the most effective means of improving the mental health of children and adolescents is by improving the ability of mainstream agencies to deliver help and support before problems become intractable' (Baring 1999: 56).

It is apparent that current referral processes are quite haphazard in enabling children and young people to access help with bereavement, and this is a key issue which needs to be addressed. It is likely that young people most in need of bereavement services may be the least likely to be referred to them – for example, vulnerable young people living in disadvantaged areas.

The literature review again reveals the extent to which different disciplines, and different methodologies, appear to be used by various protagonists in quite selective ways to promote particular points of view. It is apparent, however, that we know very little about many important aspects of how to help young people in ways that they will find appropriate and effective, given that the existing research is very largely based on people who are already in contact with services. We have very little evidence about how bereaved young people generally view their needs and how they may (or may not) cope in the absence of such services or interventions. We do not know how many more young people may be struggling to 'cope', like Neville, or facing increased vulnerability, like Brian, even years after a significant bereavement.

PART 3
Conclusions

6 Knowledge, 'meaning', and interdisciplinarity

Introduction

> ... it is not all confusion; there is such a thing as morality, even if it is inevitably contested, such a thing as knowledge, even if it is not absolute; there are power differences between people that can be creative as well as destructive.
>
> (Craib 1994: 186)

In this final chapter, I[1] will begin by considering the discussion so far, seeking to establish what conclusions we may draw from the existing evidence about young people's experiences of bereavement and loss. While some conclusions may indeed be possible, it is also apparent that the existing evidence is contradictory, complex and inadequate. Accordingly, I will then turn to consider how the work might be taken forward, and, in particular, how we might promote a dialogue across the existing disciplinary divisions that characterize and impoverish the existing research evidence. Towards this end, I will undertake an extended diversion to consider whether a focus on 'meaning' might have some real benefits to offer, although such a focus first requires us to have some clarity about what we mean by 'meaning'. Finally, I will return to our substantive focus on young people and bereavement, to examine the possible benefits of a focus on 'meaning' for furthering our knowledge about this very real and everyday issue.

Difference and continuity

In this project, we set out to take an overview of research on bereavement and young people, to consider where the boundaries and contours of the current literatures are drawn. In doing so, we hoped to point to the possibilities of finding connections and continuities with other bodies of work, while

---

[1] The use of the first person singular here is used to indicate that the arguments made in this chapter are those of Jane Ribbens McCarthy alone. However, the first person plural is still used in this chapter when the argument is drawing on the project as a whole, which has been a collaborative effort in various ways.

reflecting on where and why differences and breaks occur within the social and organizational contexts of knowledge production. This was an ambitious endeavour, and we may well have fallen short on the task we set ourselves. At the same time, it has been an exciting way to work, and we have felt intrigued and challenged by the links that can be suggested between varied theoretical perspectives and empirical bodies of work. It has also been regrettable to realize the ways in which much existing debate is quite partisan and partial, which then feeds into the empirical research output.

An implicit assumption running throughout the project has been a view of knowledge as necessarily socially produced, in that it is always situated and partial, mediated by language, and dependent on the questions we choose to ask, the conceptual and theoretical assumptions by which we frame them, and the strengths and limitations of the methodologies by which we seek to answer them. This is not to take a totally relativist view of knowledge, and, indeed, it should by now be apparent that we regard it as extremely important to find robust ways of determining the rigour and standing of any particular piece of research, as we seek to build a knowledge base that may be relevant to the needs of our particular cultural communities at this particular socio-historical juncture.

This project, of course, must also be viewed as part of this social production of relevant knowledge, and has its own particular strengths and limitations. Our own citing of the literature has thus also been partial and selective, as practical constraints impinged upon us. What we have sought to do, therefore, is to cover the variety of views and a substantial range of the evidence relevant to each view, rendering our conclusions about empirical evidence tentative. Maybe this is appropriate, however, given the contested and confusing nature of much of this evidence – as key writers in these areas themselves discuss. Part of the difficulty, too, is that, once we opened up the boundaries around the literature that we might discuss under the rubric of 'bereavement, loss and young people', to consider bereavement and loss more generally and their relevance to the lived experiences of young people in a more holistic way, we found the potential links with other debates and areas of academic and professional work to be multifarious.

We are also conscious of the ways in which we have ourselves reproduced some of the existing contours and limits of the literature on bereavement and young people. Most notably, the real dearth of research about young people's experiences of bereavement in the context of deaths that do not constitute a major disruption to their lives has meant that we have largely reproduced a picture of bereavement as being of wider interest only when it constitutes a *significant biographical event*. We have thus run the risk of replicating a view of bereavement as relevant only to a minority of young people, when the reality is that the vast majority report experiencing a significant bereavement in their lives by the time they reach age 16 (Chapter 1). In relation to policy issues, therefore, we have argued elsewhere (Ribbens McCarthy and Jessop 2005) for the importance of pursuing bereavement as a 'mainstream' issue that needs to be considered across the full range of services and settings with which young people are involved. The case studies presented in Chapter 3 attempted to provide new materials to help broaden our perspective on the range of deaths that may impinge on young people's everyday lives, and the impact that may result.

Additionally, however, even in relation to the existing research on bereavements that constitute a major disruption to young people's lives, we have ourselves drawn selectively on the published evidence. We have, for example, largely drawn on the empirical research evidence about parental and sibling bereavement (Chapters 3 and 4), and in the process, we have ourselves contributed to the disenfranchisement of bereavements that have received less research and theoretical attention, such as: bereavement of a peer, friend or partner; miscarriage and abortion; bereavements and losses experienced by refugees, who may be migrating from societies with quite different levels of violence and death at young ages (discussed briefly in Chapter 2); or by those with learning disabilities (Oswin 1991). As we have discussed, the empirical literature can thus be mapped by reference to *categories of loss* – parents, siblings, boyfriends and girlfriends, other close friends or peers, other relations – and by *types of death*. Some of these divisions in the literature, especially those which serve to construct perceptions of what is core and what is 'marginal', are ones that we have ourselves rather regrettably reinforced in this book, although we are very aware that an examination of that which is constructed as 'marginal' may often shed illuminating light on what is taken for granted, or assumed, within the more general research picture.

Furthermore, despite our discussion in Chapter 2 of theoretical perspectives that seek to reflect upon, and make explicit, some of the ways in which death and bereavement experiences in contemporary western societies may occur within institutional and cultural contexts that are historically and socially specific, we have found ourselves struggling to find ways to incorporate such insights in the details of the literature review. And alongside such theoretical and substantive divisions within the various relevant literatures, we have also grappled with the methodological diversity and complexity of the associated empirical research base.

Here, however, I will attempt to offer some tentative thoughts about what may be learned from the diverse materials we have considered in this project.

Conceptual/theoretical issues

The title of this book follows common practice by linking the concept of 'bereavement' with that of 'loss'. Nevertheless, the question arises as to whether it is useful to frame bereavement within a 'loss' perspective (see Chapter 2). This in itself points to issues of continuity and difference. The theoretical framework of 'loss' has the potential to find continuities with other life experiences that may help reduce any sense of difference. But not all bereavements are experienced as losses, and, in this respect, concepts of 'change' or 'transition' may have advantages. On the other hand, some bereavements may be experienced as so overwhelming they may seem quite unlike any other experience of loss.

But does the specific focus on young people in relation to bereavement lead us to identify particular issues about bereavement experiences during this part of the life course? It is apparent that any answers to this question will be heavily dependent on the ways in which we understand the teenage years, and the time trajectory we use to interpret this question.

In Chapter 2, we discussed the significance of the various ways in which the teenage years may be theorized from different disciplinary perspectives. 'Adolescence' is the key concept within the more psychologically-based approaches, drawing attention to what are theorized as 'developmental' processes and stages, often regarded as fundamentally underpinned by biological changes. While the more recent work within developmental psychology may be concerned to contextualize such theories by reference to social and cultural differences, this is not apparent in much of the work that considers bereavement issues through the lens of 'adolescence'.

More sociological approaches to young people draw attention to the teenage years as a phase within the life course trajectory, as a time of 'transition' between the socially constructed statuses of Child and Adult. From this perspective, experiences that individuals may share by virtue of their status as 'teenager' or 'young person' must be primarily understood in terms of different status categories which are *relational*, based in patterns of power that are underpinned by institutional arrangements and other features of social structure.

Commentators on the more psychological approaches may often criticize them, then, for presuming an implicit and unwarranted universalism about the processes they research, with a resulting insensitivity to, and neglect of, the ways in which individual lives occur within, and are shaped by, cultural contexts and features of social structure such as gender, class and race. This criticism seems to be very pertinent to much research on bereavement and young people, which often fails to mention the social characteristics and circumstances of the individuals being studied, let alone the implications of such characteristics for the ways in which bereavement may be experienced and understood by the individuals concerned. Professional theories and interventions, too, may similarly be critiqued for their tendency to reproduce, through their unexamined assumptions, approaches to grief that are compatible with the experiences of those white, middle-class (middle-aged?), western individuals who have felt the urge to become professionally involved in these difficult and painful areas of life, as these occur within particular societies at a particular point in historical time.

Sociological theorizing, however, is often heavily criticized for failing to take account of individual perspectives, differences and agency, leading to an overly deterministic view of life experiences. Mainstream sociologists would counter this critique by pointing to the central preoccupation of much contemporary social theory with precisely this issue of how we can understand the interconnections of social structure and individual agency. Much recent theorizing from both modernist and post-modernist perspectives has emphasized the plurality of consumer-based lifestyles available to individuals, and the consequent significance of individual choice, often leading to a questioning of the authority of 'expertise' and the relevance of 'meta-narratives' that seek to provide broad explanations of major features of social life.

Nevertheless, in the context of our interest here in bereavement, it is very apparent that this aspect of contemporary lives in industrialized western societies has been very much regarded as a matter of individual, 'private' experience that lies outside the province of sociology and social theory more broadly. At the same time, the rapid proliferation of various forms of professional expertise around grief and bereavement perhaps leads to new expectations and social regulation about what is appropriate for bereaved individuals to feel and do (Craib 1994; Walter 1999; Small and Hockey 2001). What has been very apparent, therefore, is that issues concerning bereavement and young people have been left very largely unaddressed by sociologists, who – with a very few honourable exceptions – have abandoned the whole area of bereavement and grief to the considerations of psychologists and the more individually-focused professionals.

It is apparent that there are different contributions and different gaps between the various disciplines, even while the divisions between the disciplines may themselves be a matter of sociohistoric contexts (Moran 2002). Psychology, counselling, medically-based and social work literatures have thus been strong on empirical evidence, and on theorizing individual grief processes (though these may be strongly debated), but weaker on theorizing at the broader level of the meanings of contemporary experiences of death and bereavement in a cultural context, and the social processes that contextualize the bereavement experiences of individual young people. In answering the question of whether there are particular issues about bereavement in the adolescent years, psychologists and clinicians have been concerned to demarcate normal and pathological/complicated grief, and to consider how to operationally identify such demarcations during the teenage years (e.g. Birenbaum 2000; Wheeler and Austin 2000). Some writers have also suggested that bereavement may be particularly complex and raise specific issues for individuals in their teenage years who are dealing with particular adolescent developmental tasks (Raphael 1984; Balk 1996; Fleming and Balmer 1996).

Notions of normal and pathological/complicated grief are important for practical considerations concerning allocation of resources, whether in terms of finances or clinicians' time. Such distinctions are associated with clinical judgements concerning which individuals may be expected to benefit from expert interventions. Other writers, however, suggest that normal grief itself should be regarded as 'complicated' (Attig 2002), and some professionals argue that significant bereavements of any sort pose emotions and challenges that may call for counselling or other supportive interventions in a non-clinical style (Stokes *et al.* 1999; Winton 2002), while others again suggest that definitions of pathology themselves reflect the pain of the professionals (Craib 1994). But such practical decisions have significant wider consequences. As Lewis comments (2000: 15) in relation to social policy formation generally:

> ... social differences are formed in the dynamic interplay of domination and inequality and the struggle against it; between the attempt to establish the boundaries of 'the normal' and attempts to dislodge and/or explain those boundaries; between the attempts to limit the criteria of access to resources and the struggle to breach or replace those criteria.

Some of these debates also point, however, to questions of the general medicalization of bereavement in western cultures (Craib 1994). In this regard, sociologists have been strong on the general theorizing of death and dying, and the significance of the developmental of medical and psychological expertise for the regulation of individuals' lives (Rose 1989; Seale 1998), but their neglect of bereavement experiences leaves a significant theoretical and empirical lacuna. This is despite the clear potential relevance of wider sociological work about historical processes of civilization (Elias 2000) leading to the development of expectations of the management of emotions in contexts of social settings that are understood as public or private (Ribbens McCarthy and Edwards 2002). Sociological work has thus been very weak on empirical work, and on theorizing individual bereavement experiences. We would contend that such a split between the contributions of psychological and sociological work to our understandings of bereavement in the lives of young people, is unnecessary and is not inevitably part and parcel of these different disciplinary frameworks. Furthermore, it can be argued that the

experiences of individual bereaved young people can only be fully understood within the wider cultural and social contexts of high and post-modernity (see Chapter 2), with fundamental implications for the development of
effective policies and practices.

Methodological considerations

Alongside such broad questions of disciplinary perspectives, and theoretical
orientations, we have also sought to explicate some of the major methodological limitations of current research. In this regard, we have become aware
of the extent to which the evidence is very much driven by researchers' own
agendas, including their own beliefs about how to deal with painful issues.
There are underlying queries, then, about what draws people to work in these
areas in the first place (see Chapter 1). Such personal perspectives become a
real obstacle, however, when they lead to the widespread practice of citing
evidence selectively, and even, at times, what appears to be a total mis-citing
of existing evidence.

Furthermore, much of the existing research has been conducted in the
USA. Not only does this root it within contemporary western cultures, it also
sets it within particular cultural, policy and institutional contexts that may
not be immediately generalizable in any straightforward way to other western
societies.

Other methodological weaknesses have been examined in some detail in
relation to both qualitative and quantitative studies (see Chapters 3 and 4),
and their particular requirements for robust research design. Common to all
methodologies are issues about the nature of the samples being studied,
which is particularly difficult to rectify on such a sensitive topic and with no
readily available sampling frames providing access to the general population
of young people in the community who have experienced bereavement.
Furthermore, all research suffers from the difficulties of how to understand
the views and needs of those who do not participate in research – whether
this is because the most vulnerable people are difficult to reach, or because
'talk' and 'participation' are not major life strategies for some individuals, or
some other reason. Non-response rates in studies of bereaved young people
are generally high, and even those projects that make great efforts to obtain
'representative' national or community-based samples of young people may
under-represent the impact of bereavement if non-response occurs dis-
proportionately from more disadvantaged groups (Elliott *et al.* 1993). On the
other hand, many studies make use of opportunistic samples, seeking to
target bereaved young people specifically, which carries the danger of over-
representing bereaved young people with problems as well as those who seek
support or who value talking.

The more qualitative evidence also points to the importance of considering bereavement in a long-term perspective, and many studies point to
the ways in which its impact may not be just a short-term experience. This
then raises further methodological issues about how to study such long-term
implications. Longitudinal studies may not be the only answer here. Eth and
Pynoos (1994), for example, studied the reactions of children and young
people to witnessing the violent death of their parent, using a sample of
recently bereaved children alongside a sample of adults who had been bereaved in this way years earlier, while Bradach and Jordan (1995) obtained
retrospective accounts of bereavement over several generations among college students. The in-depth case studies produced for this book (see Chapter
3) are unusual in being able to follow the experiences of ordinary young
people over several years.

The experience of a major disruptive and difficult event, such as bereavement of a close relationship, also raises the possibility of quite opposite
reactions occurring among different individuals, with some finding new resources and strengths, while others struggle to cope at all. Such polarized
responses may, however, cancel each other out in large-scale aggregated
quantitative data sets.

Risk assessment regarding bereavement and young people

One particular feature of contemporary western culture is arguably a preoccupation with 'risk' and attempts to predict and control it, particularly in
terms of social policies and professional interventions. At the level of individual experience, life events over time may enable some individuals to feel
empowered to deal constructively and actively with the trauma of significant
bereavement both in terms of the material consequences and the development of personal meanings that provide some sense of accommodation or
even a positive outcome. For others, however, life experiences may succes-
sively disempower them, making life appear full of unpredictable and
alarming uncertainties, with a multitude of problematic consequences that
may lead to a sense of an impoverization of life choices both materially and
spiritually. Risk assessment at a generalized level was the primary focus of
Chapter 4, although the growing awareness of the complexity of causal pre-
dictions in this area has led to an increasing interest in notions of 'resilience'
and what might moderate experiences, and 'protect' individuals from what
might otherwise lead to damaging consequences.

The empirical literature on young people and bereavement, as discussed
above, can be mapped by reference to the category of loss, and the cause of
death. It can also be mapped by reference to the outcomes being considered.
On the whole, there is a marked division in the literatures between those that

focus on personal outcomes (physical and mental health) and those that are concerned with social adjustment outcomes (educational qualifications, offending, employment, early sexuality and partnering) (see Chapter 4). Social policies may take more notice of the latter, especially in relation to the commitment of resources if bereaved young people might be considered to be at risk of social exclusion. But help organizations on the ground take more notice of the former (see Chapter 5). Again, we need to distinguish between short-term risks (which may require support with regard to the emotions and transitions of significant bereavements and disrupted biographies), and long-term risks (which may be harder to identify). Some of the relevant evidence here is to be found in studies that are actually focused on divorce as a source of 'risk' in young people's lives, but the danger then is that bereavement is only used as a source of comparison, to shed light on issues of divorce (see Chapter 4). Consequently, issues concerning bereavement in its own right may not be addressed by such research.

Furthermore, the existing research base points to the complexity of the issues involved concerning the implications of bereavement for young lives, even in relation to just the one category of bereavement that has received sustained attention (i.e. loss of a parent through death). A variety of individual, family, social and structural factors all need to be considered, for example: the gender of the bereaved young person in relation to the gender of the parent who has died; social class and household resources; pre-bereavement histories; whether or not the surviving parent remarries; the nature of continuing family relationships after death; other supports available; aspects of personality; and the significance of other losses experienced. Furthermore, there can also be interactions between these sorts of variables and the nature of the loss: Worden *et al.* (1999), for example, found that gender mediated bereavement differently according to the category of loss – sibling or parent.

Thompson (2002) suggests that whether or not a particular bereavement becomes a crisis for an individual may be understood in terms of either a bereavement that is not in itself too difficult for the individual to 'manage' but that may constitute the 'last straw' in terms of difficulties that individual may be experiencing; and a bereavement that may constitute a traumatic crisis *per se*. The first of these possibilities points to the likelihood that bereavement may well be a significant risk factor for individuals within constellations of other aspects of their lives. Bereavement may thus significantly increase the vulnerability of people who may already be at risk for other reasons, or when it is followed by other problematic experiences that compound the initial loss in an incremental way that puts individuals at risk over the life course. This view is strongly supported by evidence concerning the significance of multiple deaths, and also of multiple disadvantages of various types, for negative social and mental health outcomes. In this respect, evidence on bereavement as a source of risk is very much in line with more general research on sources of risk and resilience in the lives of children and young people (see Chapter 4).

The social effects of bereavement have, however, been generally neglected, in relation to the impact on peer relationships, and the possibility of (long-term) isolation and a sense of difference. Given the significance of this issue in young people's own accounts (see Chapter 3), the extent to which young people may not talk to anyone about their experiences (see Chapter 5), and the relevance of this for some of the controversies for how to help young people (in terms of opportunities to talk and find peer group support, see Chapter 5), this is an important area for further work.

Throughout the existing research base, there has also been a real neglect of issues concerning structural and cultural differences of a variety of types (ethnicity, class, regional, or based in particular neighbourhood or family histories). In this regard, we need to be able to disentangle issues of socio-economic circumstances in households and localities, alongside individualized and institutionalized experiences of racism, classism and sexism. Research has hardly touched upon such issues in the contexts of bereavement, although issues of ethnic and faith cultures in a broad, abstracted, sense have received attention in some guides written for practitioners (see Chapters 2 and 4).

The contexts of death and bereavement in the lives of young people

In seeking to consider the general everyday contexts in which young people live their lives and deal with experiences of bereavement, we have to consider the relative powerlessness of 'youth' in obtaining information, or determining what settings they will engage with. In terms of informal social support, alongside reports of the key importance of close friends, experiences of isolation and stigma are apparent, again raising the question of whether death and bereavement are seen as marginal and a source of difference, rather than understood to be a 'normal' part of experience during the teenage years. Supportive friendships can clearly make a real difference to the bereavement experiences of young people, but peer relationships may also well add to the difficulties. The qualitative evidence concerning young people's own perspectives suggests that there are indeed few social practices available to young people to make their grief visible (see Chapter 3).

In terms of institutional policies and interventions – whether from schools or specialist bereavement organizations – the picture appears messy and haphazard, although steps have begun to be taken in the UK to map some of these and coordinate them (see Chapter 5). The heated nature of the debates about appropriate interventions is also apparent. The lines here may not so much be drawn up in terms of different disciplines, but rather in terms of different professionals and practitioners, whether clinicians or counsellors. Thompson (2002) suggests, further, that loss and grief are also seen as specialized matters, and cut off within the theoretical framework of human service professions generally. But, as Thompson also points out, we may also need to consider whether, and in what ways, any forms of intervention (from 'death and loss education', to peer support groups, to individual counselling) may undermine, or enhance, individuals' own abilities and capacities to deal with future losses and crises.

Some of these issues of social context, whether informal or institutional, may well reflect society's wider difficulties in facing death, dying and painful bereavement issues (see Chapter 2). This points to major issues about the underlying social and historical processes that have led to the contemporary 'sequestration of death', and whether and how such deep-rooted cultural attitudes may change. One implication of this, however, would perhaps point to support for the pervasive arguments that are made for the inclusion of death, bereavement, loss and change, as part of the general school curriculum. There is provision for this within UK PSHE and citizenship education, and relevant curriculum materials are available, as well as moves towards defining emotional literacy generally as an important aspect of education for life (Chapter 8). But there is little evidence that these opportunities are taken up within schools. It is also apparent that very few schools have either formal policies or trained, designated individuals in place to respond to the needs of bereaved individuals, or of general crisis situations. Several writers point to professionals' unease about their competence and willingness to work in these areas. But programmes for emotional literacy in schools also raise issues of cultural differences, in terms of what may be perceived as 'appropriate' ways to 'manage' emotions. This would point to the possibilities for new forms of institutionalized racism, classism and sexism (including the imposition of a more female-oriented approach to emotion management on males who experience other strategies of emotion management in male culture – Walter 1999). There is also evidence that substantial proportions of young people do not want schools to be involved in such 'private and personal' issues – what seems important, therefore, is for young people to be consulted and their variable views dealt with by variable responses.

Peer support groups, whether inside or outside schools, offer a promising way of enabling young people to support each other and perhaps reduce stigma, especially if set alongside the inclusion of death and loss education in the general curriculum, with links and continuities being made with other forms of difficult life experiences where appropriate. Much would depend, however, on whether or not such groups are able to build closely upon young people's own varied experiences and perceptions, rather than (perhaps even very subtly) imposing an 'expert' model of what are considered to be appropriate grief reactions and processes.

So there are various models and possibilities for how to help individual bereaved young people within mainstream services. Specialist bereavement organizations may themselves also work with different models of intervention, with some making strong moves towards the provision of universal counselling support for young people bereaved of a close family member (Stokes 2004). Nevertheless, there are others who argue that such counselling may not always be either justified or beneficial. This perspective has to be set alongside the evidence of significant levels of distress, the high levels of those young people who say they have never talked about the bereavement to anyone, and the clear evidence that some young people are significantly and directly at risk as a result of the consequences of bereavement (Cross 2002). Any overall strategy of provision for bereaved young people may require a range of supports to be available from both mainstream services and specialist bereavement organizations, with a range of possible interventions, from basic information and acknowledgement of what has happened, to peer group support, individual counselling and clinical interventions. Individual preferences for talk or activity are also recognized to vary greatly.

However, within the current literature and provision of services, issues of referral processes have not been addressed, to enable young people to know what support might be available to them if they want it. Some evidence suggests that access to services may be quite haphazard (see Chapter 5), and that front-line mainstream professionals (such as GPs, hospitals, teachers or clergy) are ill-prepared to help, or to provide routes on to other sources of support.

As a first step, we need to know more about how young people themselves experience bereavement, and deal with it in their everyday lives. We also need to establish whether or not bereaved young people themselves want more opportunities to talk or access other sorts of support provisions.

Our current knowledge base

It is apparent that, alongside important progress, there are numerous difficulties facing us in seeking to identify and understand young people's experiences of bereavement. While it has been possible to identify some interim conclusions from the existing literature, and their implications for policy and practice, it is apparent overall that there is much still to be done. The difficulties in the current literatures may be summarized as:

- The clear disciplinary and methodological divides that exist in the current evidence, with some approaches very much predominating, and other approaches largely sidelined. Furthermore, there seems to be little awareness of, and reflection upon, such divisions.

- The consequence of this is that we have very closed and self-referential circles of discussion, with little dialogue (or even, at times, respect) across the divides, along with a limitation in the sorts of questions being asked.
- The research evidence that we do have is often extremely complex and contradictory, and sometimes hotly contested.
- All of this creates a good deal of confusion for policy-makers and practitioners alike, leading to disputes about how we should assess the appropriateness of policy and practice responses.

Such a picture should not, however, lead us to neglect the strengths of what evidence we do have, and the implications for policy and practice, nor should it lead us to despair of the key contribution that research can make. Instead, I would argue, it suggests a strong obligation on researchers to find ways forward, part of which must involve a dialogue across existing academic divides, perhaps redefining some of the contours of the literature in the process. While conclusive answers may never be possible in the face of some of life's greatest imponderables (Attig 2002), the search for knowledge and understanding continues.

Finding 'meaning' in the face of chaos?

From this complex and difficult picture, how can we find a way forward, given the variety of questions being asked, the varying practical and professional needs and disciplinary and theoretical orientations by which they are being framed, and the differing methodological approaches being used to answer them? Should we accept that such variety and complexity is simply a realistic response to the immense range of human experiences and human spirit, or is there any scope for greater dialogue and understanding between the different protagonists (as they often seem to position themselves)?

But how far can we expect any sort of agreed, or confident, knowledge when even the most basic of concepts involved – including 'bereavement' itself – may be extremely difficult to operationalize or objectify? Even if we restrict bereavement to loss through death, can we establish which categories of relationships, when ended by death, 'count' as a bereavement for the individual? Clearly, the death of a stranger is not likely to constitute a bereavement, but what of the death of a neighbour, a friend, a celebrity, an ex-mother-in-law, an absent father etc. etc.? Bereavement as a concept depends on the presumption that a social relationship has been ended (or disrupted) through death or loss, entailing what Seale argues to be 'extreme damage to the social bond' (1998: 193).

It is thus not possible to 'read off' the significance of a particular bereavement from simply identifying the category of relationship involved. We have to recognize that its significance is likely to stem from two features of the prior relationship: firstly, its ramifications for the individual's position in social life – which may include all sorts of issues for personal and social identity, material well-being and wider social networks, derived from broader institutional structures and processes; and, secondly, its much more personally-experienced meaning derived from the particularistic, inter- and intra-psychic dynamics of the relationship between two specific people over time and space. Clearly these features may well be closely interrelated, as well as heavily dependent on cultural and historical context. In the context of trauma research more generally, Janoff-Bulman (1992) points to the importance of subjective perceptions in determining whether or not a particular event is experienced as traumatic, but she also suggests this is not solely a matter of perception, and advances arguments concerning the nature of events that are more likely to lead to traumatized reactions. Within this, she suggests that particular bereavements may or may not be experienced as traumatic.

It could thus be suggested, perhaps, that we might be warranted in making some assumptions within a particular cultural context that certain relationships (and hence certain bereavements) are 'objectively' likely to have greater social significance than others – for example, in the UK today, a child's relationship with her or his mother, or an adult's relationship with her or his spouse. But even this may vary greatly in individual cases, in terms of both the particularities of the individual's 'objective' life course and the way in which the individual 'subjectively' understands ('gives meaning to') the circumstances of their life and social context in which the relationship is set. And the direct, personal, 'subjective' meaning of a particular relationship will also be crucial as to whether and how it constitutes a 'significant' bereavement, or even whether it constitutes a bereavement at all. 'Bereavement' is, then, arguably an inherently 'subjective' concept for social scientific inquiry, which intrinsically requires us to incorporate attention to the 'meaning' that any death experience holds for the individual. And young people, particularly, may be experiencing a time of life when they are especially concerned with re-evaluating the meanings of their relationships and identities, which may thus be in flux.

Indeed, 'meaning' itself has been increasingly highlighted by a number of writers on the topics of death and bereavement (and trauma more generally) – from a whole range of backgrounds – as a crucial (even central) issue which researchers and practitioners alike must incorporate into their work in these areas. Some authors thus suggest (as we have seen in Chapter 2) that 'meaning' is central to our understanding of any grieving crisis and processes that follow bereavement. And even the more quantitative researchers have indicated the relevance of 'meaning' if we are to make any advances in understanding the complexities of the 'objective' data available. Furthermore, it is also argued that a focus on 'meaning' provides particular opportunities to 'see the constant interaction between circumstances and the ways we are predisposed to interpret them' (Marris 1996: 4), thus enabling inter-disciplinary insights.

For example, Robert Neimeyer is one researcher and practitioner who has – in collaboration with various colleagues – particularly focused on issues of 'meaning', both in the context of therapeutic interventions towards 'meaning reconstruction' (2000), but also across the disciplines: 'Viewed in a broad, interdisciplinary perspective, the phenomena of loss, grief and mourning are permeated with meaning' (Neimeyer *et al.* 2002: 248). It is not perhaps too surprising to hear this from a writer such as Neimeyer, with his strong interest in narrative methodologies and meaning reconstruction theory, but it is notable that some more quantitative researchers also call for a need to focus on 'meaning'. For example, we find Michael Rutter (2000: 390), a key re-searcher for the assessment of 'risk' factors in the lives of children, calling for an emphasis on 'meaning' as a way forward in trying to understand the complexities of the quantitatively-based evidence: 'It has been crucially im-portant to appreciate that the risk derives as much from the meaning at-tributed to the event as from the objective qualities of the event itself'.

From a more directly therapeutic perspective, we also find other writers suggesting that 'meaning' is central to a great range of therapeutic inter-ventions: 'all psychological therapies share a commitment to transforming the meanings that clients have attached to their symptoms, relationships and life problems' (Brewin and Power 1997: 1). And, in the context of adolescent life crises or bereavement experiences particularly, Ayers *et al.* (2003) cite a number of theoretical models that place the subjective meanings associated with such events as central. Finally, perhaps unsurprisingly, meaning has also been defined as central to spirituality across cultures: 'Spirituality refers to the ability of the human person to choose the relative importance of the physical, social, emotional, religious, and intellectual stimuli that influence him or her and thereby engage in a continuing process of meaning making' (Morgan 2002: 194).

All of this appears to promise much for the possibility that a focus on 'meaning' may provide some common ground, and I will indeed argue that a focus on 'meaning' has much to offer as a framework for theorizing and researching young people's experiences of bereavement. Such a focus on meaning can arguably cross both disciplinary and methodological divides, promoting dialogue, cross-fertilization, and even perhaps some integration, between the various bodies of literature and research that are currently quite bounded and enclosed by disciplines, theoretical perspectives and metho-dological frameworks. It might also help us to understand some of the complexities and contradictions that are found in the current evidence.

Approaches to 'meaning'

It is perhaps not surprising that I might be optimistic about the possible contribution to be gained by a focus on 'meaning' in illuminating our knowledge about young people's experiences of bereavement. As a sociologist with a long-standing interest in family issues, and experience of using qualitative methodologies, I would position most of my work as lying within an interpretivist sociological framework, drawing broadly on the perspectives of symbolic interactionism, phenomenology and ethnomethodology. Within such established sociological approaches, the 'meanings' that social actors give to their experiences are understood as crucial and inevitable elements of social processes, building on Thomas and Znanieki's famous contention that, if people define things as real, they are real in their consequences. Such meanings are developed by individuals in the course of their interactions with others, drawing creatively on the variable meanings available to them in their particular circumstances as these are shaped and constrained by cultural and material contexts. Within such a framework, 'meanings' are inevitably always present, and are not regarded as correct or incorrect, healthy or unhealthy, but as key features of social life that require our attention and understanding if we are to produce effective analyses of social situations. Such an approach to bereavement research can be exemplified in the work of Janice Nadeau (1990) who has researched family members' meanings in response to bereavement, using a social-interactionist/phenomenological approach based on the work of such sociological writers as Berger and Luckmann, and Lofland (discussed further below).

There are various such academic traditions that may be broadly described as adopting a hermeneutic approach, which put 'meaning' front stage (albeit sometimes in different ways). And it is certainly the case that 'meaning' has been much more centrally the concern of some areas of social inquiry and practice than others – though, for the present discussion, I am focusing primarily on the disciplines of psychology and sociology. In some contrast to the hermeneutic traditions, the more scientific (often quantitative) traditions in these disciplines have paid less attention to 'meaning' (and in some scientific approaches have explicitly tried to exclude issues of meaning). Some of these variations do, however, both cross-cut disciplinary divides, while also creating divisions within the disciplines themselves.

Within sociology, then, we find a number of hermeneutic theoretical approaches that are broadly labelled as 'interpretivist', for whom 'meaning' is crucial. These include Weber's historical (but still highly relevant) discussion of social action and *verstehen*, Schutz's development of phenomenological approaches and Garfinkel's elaboration of ethnomethodology. More recently, we find Ian Burkitt's discussion of interpretations and image-schemata, building on Merleau-Ponty's discussion of the field-of-being. Burkitt (1991: 191) asserts that 'activity is ... the bedrock of meaning', such that meaning is always generated in the context of the social and physical world of time and space, shaped by both power dynamics and personal creativity:

> ... a meaningful structure of the world emerges in sensible percep- tion, through what Johnson and Lakoff would call the image-sche- matic structures, which allow for the possibility of meaning ... [Merleau-Ponty] means that the very possibility of meaning that is linguistically articulated by social groups must already be present in the more archaic image-schematic structures of corporeal perception. (Burkitt 2003: 328)

Among psychologists, the label of 'constructivist' may be more re- cognizable as a marker of the more hermeneutic approaches, particularly rooted in the work of George Kelly on personal construct theory, but also more recently, for example, in the work of Ronnie Janoff-Bulman on as- sumptive worlds. Discourse approaches, while in themselves providing a wide range of theoretical and methodological possibilities that span across sociology and psychology (Wetherell *et al.* 2001), generally point to key debates about the significance of linguistic meanings, ranging from asser- tions (from outside discourse analysis) that language refers to real objects, to Foucault's emphasis on meaning as socially located and constitutive of power relations, to Derrida's view of meaning as itself intertextual. Narra- tive approaches – which may similarly cross-cut disciplines – in turn build on and intertwine with many of these various approaches in different ways, often treating Ricoeur's ideas as central, but leading on to work that spans across the divides of sociology and psychology, and extends into key areas of therapy, for example, as in the work of Neimeyer and his colleagues (see e.g. Neimeyer 2002).

There is, then, a huge array of hermeneutic approaches across both so- ciology and psychology that treat 'meaning' as central to social inquiry and practice. Within more scientific, perhaps positivist, approaches, on the other hand, 'meaning' may well be treated as something to be 'ruled out' of the picture, or 'controlled for' as a variable in statistical analysis. However, I have found few writers within this tradition who explicate what they mean by 'meaning'. The psychologist, Mackay, is one exception here. Drawing on the work of Petocz, Mackay treats 'meaning' as having two primary sources of relevance within a realist ontology and epistemology. Firstly, meanings may be linguistic/symbolic, that is they are referential, based in the relationships between people and real objects, and feeding into the categories and classi- fications used in social inquiry, which may be the basis for truth claims. Secondly, meanings may also be experiential, indicating motivational salience for a person's particular set of interests and related beliefs, and with consequences for psychological processes. But, while Mackay welcomes the 'return of meaning to central place in psychology' (2003: 364), he is concerned that this may be associated with a belief that meaning is not open to 'objective scientific investigation'. Mackay's position, which is set out as being diametrically at odds with a more constructivist one, is that 'meaning is part of the objective, determinate world and thus in principle open to systematic examination' (p. 366).

In Mackay's discussion, this is possible because the causes of (experiential) meaning are rooted in motivations which depend on evolutionary explanation, rather than the 'autonomous creation of persons' (2003: 371). And with regard to linguistic/symbolic meaning, while meaning is argued to arise in relation between persons and objects, Mackay wants to argue (p. 369) that such objects have an independent and objective reality, making the *a priori* assumption that person and object are indeed separate: 'The definition of an object or event, what makes it a particular thing, is independent of the relations into which it enters; either that, or it cannot enter into a relation because the relation is already (impossibly) within it'. It is not clear here whether Mackay intends to suggest that definitions and meanings are separate issues, with definitions somehow occurring outside of the human context, while meanings occur in the relation between persons and objects (and would thus appear to be intrinsically social). Overall, however, his account does seem to require a clear distinction between the more subjective phenomena of experiential meaning, and the more objective phenomena of linguistic meaning.

The meaning of 'meaning'

While I thus find Mackay's particular stance on a scientific approach to 'meaning' unconvincing and unclear, this does not mean to say that all 'objective' analysis and study of meaning is impossible. While meanings may always involve human interpretation, this does not mean to say that they are always arbitrary or unstable. Indeed, social life would be almost impossible if they were. To regard all meanings as necessarily requiring human interpretation does not therefore preclude the attempt to study them using quantitative scientific methods (as Rutter suggests), nor the endeavour to operationalize them as a basis for studying them (whether through quantitative measurement or more qualitatively). It is always the case, however, that before we can operationalize a concept in order to study it, we have to have a clear understanding of what we take it to 'mean' – in this case, the meaning of 'meanings'. And, in this regard, there would appear to be a widespread tendency for writers in this area to develop a dual approach to the concept of 'meaning', which largely – though not always entirely – seems to centre on a distinction between meaning as 'sense' and meaning as 'purpose' or 'value'.[2] And this distinction, in turn, perhaps encompasses approaches to 'meaning' as both cognition and emotion, which Carlsen (1988) argues to be intrinsically interlinked.

Meaning in terms of 'sense' thus points to the question of valid content, information or reference. However, even this quite limited meaning of 'meaning' raises the possibility that, if there is no sense to them, then phenomena have no significance – as, for example, when someone asserts that dreams have no meaning. Now clearly, in the case of bereavement, which on the one hand refers to a relationship that does have (personal) significance (or it would not constitute a bereavement in the first place), but on the other hand might refer to a death that is taken to be without 'meaning' in terms of being without sense or valid content, we might indeed find a fundamental source of contradiction and confusion. At a psychic and emotional level, a death might be felt to be highly significant, but an absence of perceived social or existential 'meaning' for the death might suggest that it is without significance. Hence, perhaps, Seale's (1998) contention that death has the potential for 'meaningless chaos'.

'Sense' thus requires there to be some sort of 'reference' for a concept, which may be built around perceptions of various kinds (through our faculties, our mental awareness, moral discernment or everyday judgement). But 'sense' can itself also involve an element of 'reason' or 'purpose', while the notion of 'common sense' points to issues of any generality or consensus in terms of what makes 'sense'. 'Meaning' can also thus point to questions of the significance of phenomena in terms of 'purpose', however that is understood. Both issues of 'sense' and 'purpose' may thus be regarded as crucial features of 'meaning', which in combination raise possibilities (of various kinds) of the 'significance' of the particular phenomena under discussion.

This dual meaning of 'meaning', as sense and purpose, is indeed prevalent among various writers who focus on 'meaning' as a key aspect of bereavement, albeit with some subtle, if important, variations. Davis *et al.*, for example, refer to the distinction made by Janoff-Bulman and Frantz between meaning-as-comprehensibility and meaning-as-significance: 'Meaning-as-comprehensibility refers to the extent to which the event *makes sense*, or fits with one's view of the world (for example, as just, controllable and non-random) whereas meaning-as-significance refers to the *value or worth* of the event for one's life' (Davis *et al.* 1998: 563, emphasis added). Davis *et al.* themselves distinguish meaning as *sense-making* and as *benefit-finding*, with

---

[2] Including Mackay's distinction between referential and experiential meaning, discussed above.

the former focused on finding some predictability in the environment and the latter on finding some personal value.

Nevertheless, as Davis *et al.* point out in a later paper (2000), even where the concept of 'meaning' is clearly explicated, operationalizing the concept for empirical research can lead to considerable confusions in practice. And, indeed, such confusions seem to work their way into their own research. In seeking to study the meanings of bereavement experiences, their research assumes that meanings are conscious and explicit, and can be verbalized. This approach cannot therefore include non-verbal meanings, nor implicit meanings. What is more, in their approach to 'meanings', it is possible for meaning to be absent from an individual's view of bereavement, while 'meaning' may be something that bereaved people may need to 'make' or 'find'. Nevertheless, the empirical complexity deepens when we find that, while individuals may be categorized by Davis *et al.* as having 'failed to find any sense' in their bereavement, among those categorized as having 'made sense', this 'sense' may indeed include the notion that it is in fact 'senseless'.

This work exemplifies the ways in which there may be methodological confusion alongside assumptions about the meaning of 'meaning', assumptions that are not made explicit and may not be shared by other writers who are concerned with 'meaning'. Thus some theoretical perspectives – as discussed earlier – may take the view that 'meaning' is always present in some way or another in individual's interactions and verbal and non-verbal behaviours. Thus, while in the research of Davis *et al.* people may be understood to have 'failed' consciously and linguistically to make sense of bereavement, a more phenomenological approach would regard sense-making as an almost inevitable feature of the social (inter)actions of bereaved persons in their everyday lives in context, although the 'sense' here might not be linguistically or consciously articulated.

For interdisciplinary dialogue to be possible, then, we need to explicate such assumptions. And if we turn to the broad academic literature of social inquiry, we find a number of further questions and possible answers concerning issues of meaning, and these questions and answers are embedded in a variety of theoretical and disciplinary frameworks, such as:

- Q. Where are meanings located?
  A. In language, in embodied behaviour or actions, in symbols and/or in objects themselves.
- Q. How are meanings known?
  A. Through empathy and understanding, and/or through an objective analysis of the context or whole in which they are located.
- Q. How are meanings derived?

A. From evolution, from sociocultural context, and/or from autonomous agency.
- Q. What is the general significance of 'meanings'?
  A. In their consequences (e.g for social interactions, spiritual
  discernment or mental health), and/or in the (arguably) constitutive nature of meanings for creating (social) realities in the first
  place.

Evaluating meanings?

Within the work on bereavement that particularly considers issues of
'meaning', it is perhaps the last of these questions that generates some of
the most obvious sources of difference between various writers. It may thus
be crucial to distinguish between those writers who seek to study and
analyse meanings in order to be able to develop effective interventions, and
those who seek to develop a more effective analysis of meanings as key
social and personal phenomena, without any (immediate) expectation of
intervention.

At the individual level, an orientation to interventions inevitably connotes an evaluative framework on which to base such activities. Such an
evaluative framework may be derived from meaning as sense or as purpose.
Thus it may be considered desirable that the individual is able to develop a
coherent narrative by which to make 'sense' of the death and bereavement, so
that social life can be maintained. It may also be considered desirable to be
able to articulate some existential answers (Neimeyer 2000; Thompson 2002)
and/or some sense of benefit from the death and bereavement, which seems
to imply finding some sense of 'purpose' in the bereavement for it to have
meaning (although see Craib 1994 for an alternative view from a psychoanalytic perspective). Whether the search for meaning here implies either
sense or purpose, these approaches are both oriented to 'helping' the bereaved individual, whether towards emotional well-being, better mental
health, the restoration of social life or spiritual growth. Additionally, for some
writers the spiritual search for meaning can extend further, towards a *moral
obligation* to find 'meaning' (Bowman 2004).

In our present context, it is crucial to bear in mind that experiences of
bereavement, as we have argued throughout, might raise significant issues of
meaning that may or may not necessarily entail suffering (e.g. see the case
studies in Chapter 3). But at a rather more general sociological level, Wilkinson (2005) argues for the importance of an attention to 'meaning' as a
central feature of his project of reviewing the possibilities of a sociological
analysis of, and contribution to, the 'problem of suffering'. Wilkinson thus
argues that sociologists have neglected the experience of suffering, but can

perhaps contribute, firstly, an analysis of how social structures and social change may shape the generation/intensification/forms of human suffering, and, secondly, an understanding of the ways in which sociocultural interpretations of suffering can generate widely differing meanings, some of which may contribute to an understanding of suffering as part of a wider or narrower picture, as more or less visible to others, and a greater or lesser source of empathy. At the same time, he explores the ways in which various writers have sought, and failed, to 'make sense' of suffering, with some arguing that what is needed is a disciplinary and paradigm shift in social analysis, others concluding that it is a key part of suffering that it is literally 'unspeakable', 'unsharable' and 'senseless', while others again seek to recognize *both* its unspeakable nature, alongside the coexisting need for social analysis (Arendt 1968, 1973 discussed by Wilkinson 2005). All of which points to the central difficulty of finding a 'content' or 'reference' for the meaning of suffering, for social analysis as much as for individual sufferers.

Nevertheless, Wilkinson's discussion passes on rather seamlessly to the possibility that it is not only 'sense' that is being sought in suffering, but 'purpose' in terms of 'positive meaning' (p. 41), since the senselessness of suffering requires that it should be '"fought against"' (Ricoeur 1995 quoted by Wilkinson 2005: 43). This resonates with Morgan's assertion (2002: 195) that 'Since the person is a meaning-seeking being, spiritual pain is produced when one has the sense that his/her life is meaningless'.

However, what is apparent is that much of this discussion of the social and philosophical analysis of pain or suffering takes place with very little empirical evidence on the actual experience of suffering. In this respect, it is perhaps instructive to bear in mind the empirical work of Davis *et al.* (2000) that shows that not all bereaved individuals initiate a search for meaning, and Nadeau's (1990) empirical work that shows how, for some, the meaning of suffering (through bereavement) may be articulated precisely through the sense that it is 'meaningless'. As Gillies and Neimeyer (2006) propose, a search for meaning may depend on whether, or how far, the death challenges the bereaved person's pre-existing meaning structures.

This points to a key issue concerning how we are to assess the significance and meaning of 'meaninglessness'. Does an indication of meaninglessness suggest something problematic about an individual's response to bereavement? How are we to interpret a young person's struggle to come to terms with the accidental death of a peer or a person's statement that the death of their loved one does not make any sense to them? Does this necessarily imply that there they are not bringing any sort of framework of reference to bear, or are they rather communicating that the death has no sense of purpose for them? Can meanings ever really be absent? Does 'meaninglessness' constitute a framework of meaning in itself? And is 'meaning' an inevitable, ever-present feature of social interaction?

Social researchers who are not oriented towards interventions in bereavement might want to consider 'meanings' without an explicitly therapeutic frame of reference (as with our analysis of the 'mundane', everyday meanings of bereavement for our teenage case studies in Chapter 3). At this point, we find some potential for common ground between those using more hermeneutic/qualitative and more scientific/quantitative approaches, in the goal of incorporating the 'meanings' of bereaved people without evaluating these. When Rutter (2000) thus suggests that we need to include a consideration of 'meaning', this is in order to build more effective statistical models, since the meaning of events for the individual may be crucial to an understanding of such phenomena as risk and resilience. And when Nadeau investigates 'families making sense of death' (1990), she is not arguing that this is necessary for their mental health, but instead is seeking to explicate the social construction of joint realities between family members, even though in her later work (2002) she does seek to draw out the implications for interventions. In her original research endeavour, she draws on some classic works of interpretive sociology, which emphasize social life as a joint construction between individuals in interaction, seeking to 'make sense' of their life experiences. From this perspective, meanings are not right or wrong, nor better or worse, they just refer to the ways in which people operate in social life. It is thus possible for Nadeau to include a category in her analysis by which people make sense of death by understanding it as 'meaningless', without implying that this represents either a spiritual or mental health crisis or deficit.

Nevertheless, as Walter (1999) points out, some other classical sociological theorists, such as Durkheim (as well as contemporary writers like Marris 1996), have indeed been concerned to identify features of social life that are more or less 'healthy' for society, by which a lack of meaning (in the form of anomie, or normlessness) could be seen to be deleterious to both the individual and to society as a whole. Wilkinson (2005) similarly argues that all three of the classical 'founding fathers' of sociology (Marx, Weber and Durkeim) were centrally concerned to analyse, and ultimately to alleviate, the human suffering they saw as generated by modern society, whether in terms of the bodily and psychic suffering of the proletariat under capitalism (Marx), the inner experience of loss of meaning under increasing rationalization and bureaucratization (Weber), or the enhanced possibility of loneliness and anomie that may accompany the increased division of labour (Durkeim). Indeed, Wilkinson (2005: 45) argues that it is the intractability of human suffering that acts as a 'vital component of processes of cultural innovation, political reform and social change', so again pointing to a sense of purpose in (generalized) suffering.

Thus, of course, the distinction between evaluative and non-interventionist social enquiries is in many ways quite artificial (even though important and useful), being a matter of degree, and of orientation. Not only may apparently 'neutral' sociological analyses of anomie or bureaucratization be taken to indicate individual and social difficulties, but apparently 'neutral' psychological research concerning people's attributions of positive meaning to their lives may also be found to relate to positive and negative affect and various types of social and personal problems (discussed by Brewin and Power 1997). Indeed, the key role of 'meaning', or finding some sense of purpose, was famously identified many years ago by Frankl as crucial to understanding the ways in which individuals may survive extreme suffering and hardship (in the form of concentration camp experiences in World War II), while for Weber, arguably the central concern of his sociological endeavour was with 'the possibility of establishing and sustaining a "meaningful" existence under conditions of modernity' (Wilkinson 2005: 56). Hence Walter's observation (1999: 125) that 'The democratization of grief, like the democratization of marriage, may be an advance in freedom, but the flipside is an increase in chaos, anomie and uncertainty'.

'Meaning' as a basis for dialogue?

Overall, then, it seems clear that 'meaning' is a widely used concept among both researchers and practitioners in the area of bereavement. For some, 'meaning' is the core concept for understanding bereavement, while for others it is not so central, but is nevertheless a concept that has to be incorporated into any model that seeks to understand and explain bereavement experiences. As a concept and theoretical focus, 'meaning' provides much scope for dialogue and even integration between the different approaches to bereavement, including across the quantitative/qualitative methodological divide. This is not the place to begin such a dialogue or integration, but perhaps the discussion here can encourage some clarity as a basis for any such conversations or debates.

From the discussion above, we can perhaps summarize the different meanings of 'meaning' under certain key headings, as involving the following.

Ontological differences between hermeneutic and scientific approaches. Does 'meaning' involve fixed points of reference that have a reality of their own (Mackay's argument), or does it involve the social construction of reality through a process of sense-making through individual agency and through social interaction? I remain unconvinced that 'meaning' can exist outside of human interpretation, and it may be that we have to conclude that it is not possible to reconcile such divergent perspectives on the 'reality' of meaning.

Conceptual differences – is meaning cognitive, and is it necessarily linguistic? Does it necessarily have to be conscious and explicit? Does it necessarily entail a sense of purpose? Can it ever actually be absent? Does it reside in the individual or in social interactions?[3] All of these stances may well be relevant at times, but such conceptual differences may require us to make some really explicit and conscious choices about our focus of concern at any one time, depending on the aims of any particular study or analysis.

Methodological differences – do we want to 'fix' meanings into measurable or recordable entities that can be empirically studied, either quantitatively, to be used to build statistical models for causal explanations, or qualitatively, to be explored and described through a process of empathy, interpretation or *verstehen*?[4] Do we need to research meanings at the level of individual cognitions or behaviours, or as aspects of group interactions and processes? It seems likely that all of these methodologies will have their particular contribution to make to our studies of bereavement.

Evaluative differences – does meaning entail a moral obligation to respond to the existential and spiritual challenges of life, death and suffering? Is it necessarily advantageous for mental health? Is it therefore to be evaluated as a requirement for spiritual and mental health, and a possibly crucial focus for intervention? Or is it something to be approached more neutrally, as an intrinsic feature of the ways in which people frame their lives in interactions with others? Again, we may find value in all of these approaches, but need to be clear about what we are trying to achieve in any particular analysis or study of bereavement.

Between them, these differences point to some of the most fundamental philosophical debates about the nature of 'truth' and how to verify knowledge (through correspondence or consensus). Furthermore, such questions point to further political issues concerning the power of knowledge claims and of 'expertise' (Ribbens McCarthy forthcoming). There are some who reject the possibility of the integration of the different meanings of 'meaning'. Writers such as Mackay would make science paramount, while others, such as Wilkinson (2005: 45), suggest that we need to reject the scientific approach altogether:

> ... a sociological response to human suffering may be conceived to require that we amplify unsettling questions of meaning and morality ... that we make abundantly clear the terminal failure of

---

[3] It is apparent, for example, in Gillies and Neimeyer's (2006) recent work towards the development of a model of meaning reconstruction in bereavement, based as it is in constructivist psychology, that meaning is assumed to be cognitive and to be located in individuals – although these authors do identify this limitation as a priority for future research.

[4] But note Stone's (2004) argument that madness – to which bereavement is often likened – may pose enormous difficulties to effective communication in any format.

understanding that takes place under the attempt to render the cultural grammar of suffering accountable to the rationality of scientific analysis.

Nevertheless, despite such possibilities for deep differences of view, some writers in recent years have taken a more optimistic view towards interdisciplinarity. In relation to psychotherapies, for example, Brewin and Power argue (1997: 1) for the possibility of a theoretical integration 'in terms of processes of meaning transformation'. Others have built on this idea creatively, seeking to develop approaches that might be seen to span some of the existing divisions (particularly prevalent since the 1960s) that occur around hermeneutic versus scientific methodologies, explanations understood as causality versus understanding, and theories based in biological versus sociocultural accounts.

Bolton and Hill (1997: 17), for example, while acknowledging that their (biologically and culturally based) approach may make 'the scientific mind uncomfortable', argue for the value of the cognitive-behavioural semantics paradigm in psychology, as a scientific approach that depends on 'meaning' in terms of ' "information" carried by mental or cognitive states', such that 'Causal explanations in biopsychological science become increasingly specific, up to and including, in the case of human beings, explanations in terms of the "personal meanings" of events and actions' (p. 22).

The potential relevance of such an approach to issues of bereavement can be seen, perhaps, when Bolton and Hill (1997: 24) discuss the various forms of possible 'disruption' in an individual's life, and the need to understand such disruption in terms of:

> ... what it means to the person as a whole, how he or she adapts to it, and makes sense of it. What appears as 'symptoms' will probably be for the most part the result of meaningful adaptations to the underlying problem, and the causal models which form the basis for ... [intervention] ... will largely invoke intentional, meaningful causation.

These writers acknowledge that such an approach cannot bridge all the divides between science and hermeneutics, which, they suggest, 'are different enterprises with a creative tension between them' (p. 25). Nevertheless, they also argue that a science without 'meaning' cannot account for behaviour, while a hermeneutics of meaning without scientific causality leaves the empirical study of 'meaning' stranded and unable to build models of how, for example, childhood adversity may have adult sequelae.

And similarly, though working with a different methodology, Neimeyer's discussion of narrative approaches spans the differences between objectivity and subjectivity. As we saw in Chapter 3, his approach thus includes the view of narratives as external (i.e. accounts of actual events and circumstances, which may be seen as objective), as well as internal (i.e. subjective accounts of emotional and experiential responses to events), and reflexive (i.e. narratives that seek to 'analyse, interpret and make meaning of an event') (2002: 53). Raskin and Neimeyer (2003) also suggest that their constructivist approach converges in important ways with Mackay's perspective on 'experiential meaning' (as discussed earlier) – even while they suggest there may be limits to the possibilities of reconciling such constructivist approaches with Mackay's realist ontology.

Overall, the widespread acceptance of a need to incorporate an attention to 'meaning' is very striking in bereavement research, perhaps suggesting that alongside the continuing tensions around ontology, theorizing, methodology and evaluation, respectful and creative dialogue across disciplinary and methodological divides might be enhanced through a shared attention to 'meaning'. Such tensions may demand clarity not only to promote dialogue across disciplines and methodologies, but also to recognize where there are limits to this, not only because there may be fundamental disagreements, but also because there may be different questions being asked for different purposes. But a concern with the lived experiences of young people who have been bereaved does perhaps impose a pressing obligation on us to work towards such dialogue, integration and clarity, as well as providing a very relevant focus for thinking about what may be required to extend the scope for interdisciplinary knowledge.

The 'meaning' of young people's experiences of bereavement

I would thus argue for the centrality of 'meaning' for the study and analysis of young people's experiences of bereavement, as being the most sophisticated and productive route forward in the face of the complex and contradictory evidence we have available to us. Furthermore, 'meaning' can arguably act as a 'hinge' between the public and private faces of such bereavement experiences, requiring us to pay attention both to their experiential qualities – qualities that may be quite unique to any particular individual – and to their occurrence in embodied social interactions and in social contexts as these occur across time and space, shaped by personal creativity as well as by power and material resources. Within both quantitative and qualitative approaches, then, we also have to recognize that the meanings of bereavement are partly dependent on the public/private discourses of grief available (Riches and Dawson 2000) (see Chapter 2). The bereavement experiences of young people thus need to be understood as both an individual experience of loss and change, shaped by the personal meanings this experience holds for each one within their life course overall, and as embedded in the wider in-stitutionalized framework of 'youth' and the ways in which this framework may shape, and be shaped by, such personal meanings. We can thus consider the potential contribution that a focus on 'meaning' may provide across disciplines and across methodologies at conceptual, methodological and theoretical levels.

The contribution of 'meaning' for conceptual issues

I have argued above that bereavement itself intrinsically requires attention to the 'meaning' a relationship holds for the individual. Additionally, we saw in Chapter 2 how some writers suggest that the grief experience can be centrally understood as a crisis of meaning. We have also noted how the topics of bereavement and youth share common concepts in terms of being theorized as 'transitions' and as sources of 'disruption', such that the conjuncture of the two may be viewed as a double jeopardy. And, as Parkes suggested many years ago now, such psychosocial transitions involve major challenges of meaning 'to basic assumptions about one's nature, needs, goals and sources of support. Bereavement, Parkes suggested, consists of the difficult and painful process of abandoning long-held assumptions and adopting new and more appropriate ones' (Brewin and Power 1997: 11).

Disruption, likewise, may be conceptually understood as fundamentally concerned with a loss of individual meaning (posing a threat to one's bio-graphical narrative – Walter 1999 – or to one's identity – Riches and Dawson 2000) and/or about a challenge to the socially constructed and in-stitutionalized meanings that frame what are considered to be 'normal' or 'typified' (Schutz 1954) everyday social interactions.

The contribution of 'meaning' for empirical and research issues

Throughout our review of the empirical research findings in Part 2, we stressed the numerous areas in which bereavement seems to raise contra-dictory implications for different individuals, families and communities. We have thus seen how bereavement may be associated with depression and lowered self-worth, or with a sense of new strength and self-esteem; with a renewed commitment to do well educationally and succeed in gaining qua-lifications, or with a loss of motivation and concentration, a decline in con-fidence and a failure to take up opportunities in higher education; with a tendency to engage early in sexual activity and partnering, or with a hesitation and postponement of involvement in intimate adult relationships; with a renewed strength and positive valuing of one's family relationships or with a sense of alienation, conflict and outright abuse within a changed family context; with the additional burden of stigma and bullying from one's peers, or with an experience of the immense support that can come from close friendships. Such polarized and contradictory tendencies may perhaps reflect the ways in which the human spirit may respond to pain and suffering, through the different ways in which we may understand profound life events, leading to a new search for meaning, or to a profound disruption of meaning, in whatever sense we are using 'meaning'.

An attention to meaning might, therefore, help to account for some of the complexity and contradictions of the quantitative research evidence (see Chapter 4). In order to advance such research, we need the development of more complex theoretical models, along with the use of sophisticated statistical methods, in combination with insights from more qualitative methods. Such models need to incorporate aspects of social structure, informal social contexts, and individual characteristics and life events. Meanings are implicated in all of these, not only at the individual intra-psychic level, but also in the ways in which other social features are understood by, impinge on, and are in turn shaped by, individuals. Additionally, social and cultural 'meanings' are crucial aspects of the interpersonal events and processes as these occur within, and are shaped by, social interactions and social structures: 'Because constructions of meaning represent the history, understanding and relationships of a culture, as well as the individual organization of experience, an analysis in terms of meaning connects personal and social processes better than the language of feeling, which has no collective counterpart' (Marris 1996: 122).

In these regards, narrative methodologies also have much to offer in terms of capturing the interplay of processes of culture, social and family contexts, social structure, and personally experienced emotion and meaning-making. In this sense, they link with the more complex theoretical models being developed in conjunction with structured methodologies. Theoretically, narrative approaches can enable us to ask whether major bereavement is usefully understood as a process of biographical disruption, a threat to identity, and/or another example of the demands imposed by the reflexivity of high modernity. In the latter regard, we may point to the consequent loss of ontological security, the role of social institutions in mediating disorder (Walter 1999) and the significance of the embodiment of bereavement – as the boundary between life and death, body and self, nature and culture – a reminder of our own embodiment (see Seale 1998).

But narrative constructions may also be used as a form of therapeutic intervention, in which a major task of grief processes is understood in terms of the necessity of reframing individual life-course narratives to take account of the disruption, both practically and existentially. While this approach thus has diverse potentials (which would be further enhanced if it were not so dependent on talk or written communication – though see also Rigazio-Di-Gilio 2001 for a narrative approach based on videography), yet again we often find an absence of dialogue between various literatures, such that potentially fruitful links may be missed across these various areas of theoretical and professional work. But overall it is clear that a range of qualitative approaches – including narrative, discourse, ethnographic and clinical work – need to be brought to bear when researching bereavement as a feature of the lives of young people in general (see Chapter 3), if we are to have any real understanding of how these events occur and are experienced in everyday lives in social contexts shaped by space and time.

A further prominent theme at the level of young people's own perceptions is that of the ways in which grief may continue to play its part in their lives over long periods of time, as their life trajectories unfold and the meaning of the bereavement comes to be reworked and re-evaluated. This was very apparent in the case studies presented in Chapter 3, drawn from a general longitudinal research database of in-depth interviews with young people in various locations in the UK over a period of several years. These case studies point to the significance of understanding any particular bereavement in the context of the individual biography as well as the meanings by which these biographies are interpreted. Furthermore, the content of these case studies points to the potential significance of bereavement even when it does not constitute a source of major life disruption. They also suggest the possibilities of individuals developing their own 'coping mechanisms', but also the ways in which young people's struggles to deal with a major bereavement over time may be lost from the view of those around them. Together the case studies point to major sources of continuities and differences regarding young people's experiences of bereavement.

Overall, it is apparent that both qualitative and quantitative research, and their associated theoretical models, need to pay rigorous attention to:

- life-course biographies, as these are interpreted by the meanings ascribed to them by individuals;
- social and institutional contexts, including education systems, occupational structures, medical and bereavement services;
- the socially structured implications of race, gender, material circumstances and social class as these get played out in everyday experiences;
- peer and family relationships;
- the contexts of particular localized settings (schools, neighbourhoods etc.);

- the fact that all these issues are played out through changes and continuities over (long) periods of time.

The contribution of 'meaning' for theoretical issues

As mentioned above, a focus on 'meaning' can also enable us to consider the possibility that bereavement experiences may be significant for young people with or without major emotional or biographical disruption. As we saw with the case studies of Shirleen and Khattab, deaths can raise major challenges of meaning even when they do not necessarily constitute a disruptive 'loss' or bereavement in young people's lives. Death and bereavement may thus constitute key issues for the development of 'meaning' for both individuals and society as a whole. Our literature review has demonstrated an almost complete absence of empirical research that has considered such major themes of young people's experiences, and this is mirrored by the lack of policy and practice regarding bereavement as a mainstream issue in the lives of young people.

This points to a need to understand much more closely how young people themselves understand or 'make sense' of bereavement, whether of greater or lesser 'significance' in their lives, without taking an explicitly evaluative stance as to the need for, or desirability of, developing such meanings. Very little research has sought to do this, and it is clear that young people themselves have often felt to be without a 'voice' – that they are positioned in a way that makes it very difficult for their perspectives to be noticed or heard, either as a child in need of special 'protection', or as an adult who can speak up powerfully about her or his own needs.

We thus need much greater recognition of the prevalence and 'normality' of bereavement experiences that are felt to be significant by young people themselves. Indeed, we also need much more reliable information to be able to establish firm knowledge about the prevalence of the wide range of young people's bereavement experiences. Death and bereavement need to be recognized as a general – 'normal' – part of growing up, as young people struggle to develop meanings and to make sense of their own identities and the social worlds of which they are part. If we fail to do so, then social inquiry may serve reflexively to help re/produce social worlds in which death and bereavement are treated as invisible, rather than core social and personal issues through which 'meanings' may be challenged and developed.

Such a wide-ranging focus feeds into the recognition of variable constituent groups for consideration by social policy, including:

- the bereavement experiences of the general population of young people;
- young people who have experienced bereavement of particularly 'close' relationships;
- problematic young people who may have (hidden) experience of variety of bereavement and loss events.

At the more theoretical level, a broader understanding of a range of bereavements as these are experienced in everyday lives perhaps points to further questions that could be raised through a greater application of sociological perspectives, which – as we have noted – have made minimal contributions to empirical work in these areas. As became clear to us in searching for relevant research literatures, the concept of 'bereavement' is very heavily based in a psychological/therapeutic/medical theoretical framework and professional practices. As a term, it is rarely used by sociologists or other academic social researchers, and is not very visible in terms of social work practices and writings.[5] We thus encountered vast amounts of written materials within some academic and professional areas, alongside very slim attention from other academic areas that could, nevertheless, provide considerable potential for developing new approaches to the general area of bereavement on the one hand, and young people on the other hand, in the context of contemporary western societies. It is apparent that a wide variety of literatures have the potential at least to provide important insights, concepts, theories and empirical findings that might be fruitful.

While some of this potential is already being developed, as we have seen in our review of existing research (Part 2), much remains implicit, with links yet to be made across diverse bodies of theoretical literature. A very brief sketch points to the following sociological perspectives that might be considered in relation to the issues of bereavement in young people's lives:

- the sociology of death and dying in western contexts, and the ways in which young people's understandings and experiences of death, dying and bereavement may be understood to be shaped by these wider sociohistorical processes;
- young people and youth as a relational status of power that is both personally and institutionally defined;
- cultural studies of media treatment, exploring the ways in which death and bereavement in western societies are mediated by distant but collectivized representations, and the ways in which this may be understood with reference to young people's use of the media;

---

[5] We are indebted to Linda Nutt for helping our thinking on this issue.

- biographical approaches which might point to an understanding of bereavements experienced by young people as (potentially) major sources of narrative disruption, or, alternatively, as part of the re-current disruptions of life (see Chapter 3 and Exley and Letherby 2001);
- sources of significant socially patterned, and structurally shaped, differences in individual biographies and experiences, including gender, generation, class, ethnicity, dis/ability and locality, that draw our attention to other key features of social contexts and biographies that may relate to young people's experiences of bereavement;
- risk factors that may be seen to shape (transitions to) adult lives in various ways, understood as the outcomes of earlier family-based, childhood experiences, placing bereavement during childhood, and/or the teenage years as having a potentially significant long-term relevance for teenagers, and for transitions to adult lives;
- general work on relationships and family change, placing change, loss, death and bereavement as a potential feature of all significant relationships in the lives of young people;
- the sociology of the body, drawing attention to the ways in which western cultures understand bodies (including mortality) in parti-cular ways, and the implications of this in the context of young people's experiences;
- the sociology of time, relevant to issues of anticipatory death, but also bereavement and the challenge to linear time (Small 2001a), and young people's own understandings of time (Brannen and Nilsen 2002);
- the sociology of emotions, particularly in the context of work on historical civilizing processes, that leads to the management of emotions and an internalized surveillance of our emotional life and its expression (Small and Hockey 2001), which may raise particular issues in relation to expectations of personal moral and emotional responsibility and accountability during the teenage years;
- mortality and bereavement as the (perhaps ultimate) experience of individual 'risk', that young people may avoid, confront and chal-lenge in various ways, as they seek to manage their own life trajec-tories within the contexts of the reflexivity of high or post-modernity.

In all these perspectives, however, a focus on 'meaning' may enable work to attend to, and build upon, the current research and theoretical knowledge base, framed as these predominantly are by psychological perspectives. But the substantive attention to young people's experiences of bereavement provides a specific focus with practical urgency and theoretical challenge for researchers across the range of disciplines and methodologies. Whether our concern is to develop policies, practices and interventions to help bereaved young people, or to develop more adequate social theory, the marginality of the experiences of youth and bereavement together raise some profound questions that may provide food for thought for all of us, about our individual psychic and spiritual experiences and the nature of our social worlds.

Conclusion

We hope this review, and the questions we have raised, will help contribute constructively to theoretical, research and policy and professional debates across the wide range of academic and applied contexts where they may be relevant. But in all aspects of the experiences we have considered here – whether of academics in various disciplines, medical, therapeutic or educational professionals, or individuals voicing their perspectives – people may seek explanations and some sense of justice or morality in the face of human mortality and suffering. Young people particularly may struggle with such issues, and we have failed to listen to their experiences and perspectives. Despite abstract or generalized anxieties concerning young people's presumed capacity for disruption during their years of transition to adulthood, it is clear that the disruption of bereavement, and the particular transitions this may entail, have received little direct attention from social policy and general social theory, and may be overlooked by society generally, as too uncomfortable to contemplate.

References

Abdelnoor, A. and Hollins, S. (2004) The effect of childhood bereavement on secondary school performance, *Educational Psychology in Practice*, 20(1): 43–54.

Abrams, R. (1992) *When Parents Die*. Charles Letts and Co.

Agid, O. *et al.* (1999) Environment and vulnerability to major psychiatric illness: a case control study of early parental loss in major depression, bipolar disorder and schizophrenia, *Molecular Psychiatry*, 4(2): 163–72.

Alderson, P. and Montgomery, J. (1996) *Health Care Choices: Making Decisions With Children (Participation and Consent)*. London: Institute for Public Policy Research.

Alldred, P. and Gillies, V. (2002) Eliciting research accounts; re/producing modern subjects?, in M. Mauthner, M. Birch, J. Jessop and T. Miller (eds) *Ethics in Qualitative Research*. London: Sage.

Alldred, P., David, M. and Edwards, R. (2002) *Minding the Gap: Children and Young People Negotiating Relations Between Home and School*. London: Routledge/ Falmer.

Allen, C., Sprigings, N. and Kyng, E. (2003) *Street Crime and Drug Misuse in Greater Manchester*. Salford: University of Salford/Home Office.

Amato, P.R. (1993) Children's adjustment to divorce: theories, hypotheses and empirical support, *Journal of Marriage and the Family*, 58: 23–8.

Amato, P.R. (2000) The consequences of divorce for adults and children, *Journal of Marriage and the Family*, 62: 1269–87.

Amaya, J.F.S. (2002) How young people live and die in a violent country: Columbian case. Paper presented at the conference of the European Sociological Association, Helsinki.

Anderson, M. (1990) The social implications of demographic change, in F.M.L. Thompson (ed.) *The Cambridge Social History of Britain 1750–1950, Volume 2: The People and Their Environment*. Cambridge: Cambridge University Press.

Ariés, P. (1974) *Western Attitudes to Death*. London: Marion Boyars.

Ariés, P. (1981) *The Hour of Our Death*. London: Allen Lane.

Armstrong, D. (1987) Silence and truth in death and dying, *Social Science & Medicine*, 24(8): 651–7.

Aspinall, S.Y. (1996) Educating children to cope with death: a preventive model, *Psychology in the Schools*, 33(4): 341–9.

Attig, T. (2002) Relearning the world: making and finding meanings, in R.A. Neimeyer (ed.) *Meaning Reconstruction and the Experience of Loss*. Washington, DC: American Psychological Association.

Atwool, N. (1997) Making connections: attachment and resilience, in N.J. Taylor and A.B. Smith (eds) *Enhancing Children's Potential: Minimising Risk and Maximising Resiliency*. Proceedings of the Children's Issues Centre Second Child and Family Policy Conference 2–4 July, 1997, Dunedin: New Zealand.

Ayers, T.S., Cara, L.K., Sandler, I.N. and Stokes, J. (2003) Adolescence Bereavement, in T.P. Gullotta and M. Bloom (eds) *Encyclopedia of Primary Prevention and Health Promotion*. New York: Kluwer Academic/Plenum.

Balarajan, R. and Soni Raleigh, V. (1997) Patterns of mortality among Bangladeshis in England and Wales, *Ethnicity and Health*, 2(1/2): 5–12.

Balk, D.E. (1983) Adolescents' grief reactions and self-concept perceptions following sibling death – a study of 33 teenagers, *Journal of Youth and Adolescence*, 12(2): 137–61.

Balk, D.E. (1991a) Sibling death, adolescent bereavement, and religion, *Death Studies*, 15(1): 1–20.

Balk, D.E. (1991b) Death and adolescent bereavement: current research and future directions, *Journal of Adolescent Research*, 6: 7–27.

Balk, D.E. (1995) *Adolescent Development: Early Through Late Adolescence*. Pacific Grove, CA: Brookes/Cole.

Balk, D.E. (1996) Models for understanding adolescent coping with bereavement, *Death Studies*, 20(4): 367–87.

Balk, D.E. (2000) Adolescents, grief and loss, in K.J. Doka (ed.) *Living with Grief: Children, Adolescents and Loss*. Washington, DC: Hospice Foundation of America.

Balk, D.E. and Corr, C. A. (1996) Adolescents, developmental tasks, and encounters with death and bereavement, in C.A. Corr and D.E. Balk (eds) *Handbook of Adolescent Death and Bereavement*. New York: Springer.

Baring, T. (1999) *Bright Futures*. London: Mental Health Foundation.

Barnes, M.K., Harvey, J.H., Carlson, H. and Haig, J. (1996) The relativity of grief: differential adaptation reactions of younger and older persons, *Journal of Personal and Interpersonal Loss*, 1: 375–92.

Bauman, Z. (1992a) *Mortality, Immortality and Other Life Strategies*. Cambridge: Polity.

Bauman, Z. (1992b) Survival as a social construct, *Theory Culture and Society*, 9: 1–36.

Bauman, Z. (1997) *Postmodernity and its Discontents*. Cambridge: Polity Press.

Bauman, Z. (1998) *Postmodern Adventures of Life and Death*. London: Routledge.

Beck, U. (1992) *Risk Society: Towards a New Modernity*. London: Sage.

Beratis, S. (1991) Suicidal attempts and suicides in Greek adolescents, in D. Papadatou and C. Papadatos (eds) *Children and Death*. New York: Hemisphere.

Birenbaum, L.K. *et al.* (1989–90) The response of children to the dying and death of a sibling, *Omega: Journal of Death and Dying*, 20(3): 213–28.

Birenbaum, L.K. (2000) Assessing children's and teenagers' bereavement when a sibling dies from cancer: a secondary analysis, *Child Care Health and Development*, 26(5): 381–400.

Birtchnell (1972) Early parent death and psychiatric diagnosis, *Social Psychiatry*, 7: 202–10.

Black, D. (1978) Annotation: the bereaved child, *Journal of Child Psychology and Psychiatry*, 19(3): 287–92.

Black, D. (1991) Family intervention with families bereaved or about to be bereaved, in D. Papadatou and C. Papadatos (eds) *Children and Death*. New York: Hemisphere.

Black, D. (1993) *Highlight. Children and Bereavement*. London: National Children's Bureau.

Black, D. (1998) Coping with loss – bereavement in childhood', *British Medical Journal*, 316(7135): 931–3.

Black, D. (2002) The family and childhood bereavement: an overview, *Bereavement Care*, 21(2): 24–6.

Bode, J. (1993) *Death is Hard to Live With: Teenagers Talk about how they Cope with Loss*. New York: Bantum Doubleday.

Bolton, D. and Hill, J. (1997) On the causal role of meaning, in M. Power and C. R. Brewin (eds) *The Transformation of Meaning in Psychological Therapies: Integrating Theory and Practice*. Chichester: John Wiley.

Bor, R., Ebner-Landy, J., Gill, S. and Brace, C. (2002) *Counselling in Schools*. London: Sage.

Boswell, G. (1996a) *Young and Dangerous: The Backgrounds and Careers of Section 53 Offenders*. Aldershot: Avebury.

Boswell, G. (1996b) The needs of children who commit serious offences, *Health & Social Care in the Community*, 4(1): 21–9.

Bowie, L. (2000) Is there a place for death education in the primary curriculum? *Pastoral Care*, 18(1): 22–7.

Bowlby-West, L. (1983) The impact of death on the family system, *Journal of Family Therapy*, 5(4): 279–94.

Bowman, T. (2004) *Literary sources for meaning-making*. Presentation made to the conference, 'What Was It All About? Meaning-Making at the End of Life and into Bereavement', Portsmouth, 15 October. Organized by the Rowan's Hospice in conjunction with the University of Portsmouth and the NHS.

Bradach, K.M. and Jordan, J.R. (1995) Long-term effects of a family history of traumatic death on adolescent individuation, *Death Studies*, 19(4): 315–36.

Brannen, J. and Nilsen, A. (2002) Young people's time perspectives, *Sociology*, 36(3): 513–37.

Brannen, J., Lewis, S., Nilsen, A. and Smithson, J. (eds) (2002) *Young Europeans, Work and Family: Futures in Transition*. London: Routledge.

Brent, D.A., Perper, J., Moritz, G., Allman, C., Liotus, L., Schweers, J., Roth, C., Balach, L. and Canobbio, R. (1993) Bereavement or depression – the impact of the loss of a friend to suicide, *Journal of the American Academy of Child and Adolescent Psychiatry*, 32(6): 1189–97.

Brewin, C.R. and Power, M.J. (1997) Meaning and psychological therapy: overview and introduction, in M. Power and C.R. Brewin (eds) *The Transformation of Meaning in Psychological Therapies*. Chichester: Wiley.

Brown, J. (2002) *Young People and Bereavement Counselling: What Influences Young People in their Decision to Access Bereavement Counselling After the Death of Someone Close?* Unpublished MA dissertation Leeds: College of York St John, University of Leeds.

Bryman, A. (2001) *Social Research Methods*. Oxford: Oxford University Press.

Buchanan, A. and Ten Brinke, B. (1997) *What Happened when they were Grown Up?* York: Joseph Rowntree Foundation.

Burkitt, I. (1991) *Social Selves: Theories of the Social Formation of Personality*. London: Sage.

Burkitt, I. (2003) Psychology in the field of being: Merleau-Ponty, ontology and social constructionism, *Theory and Psychology*, 13(3): 319–38.

Burman, E. (2000) Emotions in the classroom and the institutional politics of knowledge, *Psychoanalytic Studies*, 3(3–4): 313–24.

Bynner, J. (2001) Childhood risks and protective factors in social exclusion, *Children and Society*, 15(5): 285–301.

Bynner, J., Chisholm, L. and Furlong, A. (eds) (1997) *Youth, Citizenship and Social Change in a European Context*. Aldershot: Ashgate.

Carlsen, M.B. (1988) *Meaning-Making: Therapeutic Processes in Adult Development*. New York: W.W. Norton.

Carr, D. (2000) Emotional intelligence, PSE and self-esteem: a cautionary note, *Pastoral Care*, 18(3): 27–33.

Carson, J.F., Warren, B.L. and Doty, L. (1995) An investigation of the grief counseling services available in the middle schools and high schools in the state of Mississippi, *Omega Journal of Death and Dying*, 30(3): 191–204.

Cerel, J., Fristad, M.A., Weller, E.B. and Weller, R.A. (2000) Suicide-bereaved children and adolescents, II: parental and family functioning, *Journal of the American Academy of Child and Adolescent Psychiatry*, 39(4): 437–44.

Charlton, J. (1996) Trends in all-cause mortality: 1841–1994, in J. Charlton and M. Murphy (eds) *The Health of Adult Britain, 1941–1994*, vol. 1. London: The Stationery Office.

Christ, G. H. (2000) *Healing Children's Grief: Surviving a Parent's Death from Cancer*. New York: Oxford University Press.

Clark, D.C., Pynoos, R.S. and Goebel, A.E. (1994) Mechanisms and process of adolescent bereavement, in R.J. Haggerty *et al.* (eds) *Stress, Risk and Resilience in Children and Adolescents: Processes, Mechanisms and Interventions*. Cambridge: Cambridge University Press.

Coghlan, A. (2003) Counselling can add to post-disaster trauma, *New Scientist*, June: 5.

Cohen, J. (1999) *Educating Minds and Hearts: Social Emotional Learning and the Passage into Adolescence*. New York: Teachers' College Press.

Cohen, J. (2001) *Caring Classrooms/Intelligent Schools: The Social and Emotional Education of Young Children*. New York: Teachers' College Press.

Corden, A., Sainsbury, R. and Slope, P. (2001) *Financial Implications of the Death of a Child*. London: Family Policy Studies Centre/Joseph Rowntree Foundation.

Corr, C. A. (2000a) What do we know about grieving children and adolescents? in K.J. Doka (ed.) *Living with Grief: Children, Adolescents and Grief*. Philadelphia, PA: Brunner/Mazel.

Corr, C. A. (2000b) Using books to help children and adolescents cope with death: guidelines and bibliography, in K.J. Doka (ed.) *Living with Grief: Children, Adolescents and Loss*. Philadelphia, PA: Brunner/Mazel.

Corr, C. A. and McNeil, J.M. (eds) (1986) *Adolescence and Death*. New York: Springer.

Cowie, H. (1998) Perspectives of teachers and pupils on the experience of peer group support against bullying, *Educational Research and Evaluation*, 4(2): 108–25.

Cowie, H. (1999) Peers helping peers: interventions, initiatives and insights, *Journal of Adolescence*, 22: 433–6.

Cowie, H. (2000) Peer support against bullying, *Counselling Psychology Review*, 15(4): 8–12.

Cowie, H. and Sharp, J. (1996) *Peer Counselling in Schools: A Time to Listen*. London: David Fulton.

Cowie, H., Naylor, P., Talamelli, P., Chauhan, L. and Smith, P.K. (2002) Knowledge, use of and attitudes towards peer support: a 2-year follow-up in the Prince's Trust survey, *Journal of Adolescence*, 25(5): 453–67.

Craib, I. (1994) *The Importance of Disappointment*. London: Routledge.

Cross, S. (2002) *'I can't stop feeling sad': Calls to ChildLine about Bereavement*. London: ChildLine.

Curtis, K. and Newman, T. (2001) Do community-based support services benefit bereaved children? A review of empirical evidence, *Child Care Health and Development*, 27(6): 487–95.

Davies, B. (1991) Responses of children to the death of a sibling, in D. Papadatou and C. Papadatos (eds) *Children and Death*. New York: Hemisphere.

Davies, B. (1998) *Shadows in the Sun: The Experiences of Sibling Bereavement During Childhood*. London: Routledge.

Davis, C.G., Nolen-Hoeksema, S. and Larson, J. (1998) Making sense of loss and benefitting from the experience: two construals of meaning, *Journal of Personality and Social Psychology*, 75(2): 561–74.

Davis, C.G., Wortman, C.B., Hehman, D.R. and Silver, R.C. (2000) Searching for meaning in loss: are clinical assumptions correct?' *Death Studies* 24(6): 497–542.

DeAngelis, T. (2000) School psychologists in demand and expanding their reach, *Monitor on Psychology*, 31(8): 29–32.

Demi, A.S. and Gilbert, C.M. (1987) Relationship of parental grief to sibling grief, *Archives of Psychiatric Nursing*, 1(6): 385–91.

Dent, A., Condon, L., Blair, P. and Fleming, P. (1996) Bereaved children: who cares? *Health Visitor*, 69(7): 270–1.

Department of Health (2001) *Bereavement Services Report*. London: Department of Health.

Department of Health (2004) *Government Response to House of Commons Health Committee Report on Palliative Care, Fourth Reort of Session 2003–4*. London: MHSO.

Department of Health (2005) *Survey of Bereavement Care and other Support Services*, ww.dh.gov.uk/Publicationsandstatistics/Publications/PublicationsPolicyAnd Guidance/PublicationsPolicyAndGuidanceARticle/fs/en?CONTENT_ID= 4115879&chk=tims, Accessed 10th May 2006.

Desai, S. and Bevan, D. (2002) Race and culture, in N. Thompson (ed.) *Loss and Grief: A Guide to Human Services Practitioners*. Basingstoke: Palgrave.

Dilworth-Anderson, P., Burton, L.M. and Johnson, L.B. (1993) Reframing theories for understanding race, ethnicity and families, in P.G. Boss, W.J. Doherty, R. LaRossa, W.R. Schumm and S.K. Steinmetz (eds) *Sourcebook of Family Theories and Methods*. New York: Plenum.

Doka, K.J. (ed.) (2000) *Living with Grief: Children, Adolescents and Loss*. Washington, DC: Hospice Foundation of America.

Douglas, G., Messenger Davies, M., Doughty, J. and Lloyd, E. (2004) Research on divorce, separation and family change: messages for practitioners, *Pastoral Care*, 22(4): 3–5.

Douglas, J.W.B. (1970) Broken families and child behaviour, *Journal of the Royal College of Physicians*, 4: 203–10.

Douglas, J.W.B. (1973) Early disturbing events and later enuresis, in I. Kolvin, R.C. MacKeith and S.R. Meadow (eds) *Bladder Control and Enuresis*. London: William Heinemann.

Douglas, J.W.B., Ross, J.M. and Simpson, H.R. (1968) *All Our Future*. London: Peter Davies.

Dowdney, L. (2000) Annotation: childhood bereavement following parental death, *Journal of Child Psychology and Psychiatry and Allied Disciplines*, 41(7): 819–30.

Dowdney, L., Wilson, R., Maughan, B., Allerton, M., Schofield, P. and Skuse, D. (1999) Psychological disturbance and service provision in parentally bereaved children: prospective case-control study, *British Medical Journal*, 319(7206): 354–7.

Druce, C. and Pentland, C. (2004) Feeling alone . . . in school, Paper presented to the Childhood Bereavement Network Conference, *Feeling Alone and Different*. London: 28th April.

Dyregrov, A., Gjestad, R., Wikander, A.M.B. and Vigerust, S. (1999) Reactions following the sudden death of a classmate, *Scandinavian Journal of Psychology*, 40(3): 167–76.

Edwards, R. and Aldred, P. (2000) A typology of parental involvement in education centreing on children and young people: negotiating familialisation, institutionalisation and individualisation, *British Journal of Sociology of Education*, 21(3): 435–55.

Eisenstadt, J.M. (1978) Parental loss and genius, *American Psychologist*, 33(3): 211–23.

Eiser, C., Havermans, T., Rolph, P. and Rolph, J. (1995) The place of bereavement and loss in the curriculum: teachers' attitudes, *Pastoral Care*.

Elias, N. (1985) *The Loneliness of the Dying*. Oxford: Blackwell.

Elias, N. (2000) *The Civilizing Process*. London: Blackwell.

Elliott, J. (1999) The death of a parent in childhood: a family account, *Illness, Crisis, Loss*, 7(4): 360–75.

Elliot, J., Richards, M. and Warwick, H. (1993) *The Consequences of Divorce for the Health and Well-being of Adults and Children*. Cambridge: University of Cambridge, Centre for Family Research.

Ely, N., West, P., Sweeting, H., and Richards, M. (2000) Teenage family life, life chances, lifestyles and health: a comparison of two contemporary cohorts, *International Journal of Law, Policy and the Family*, 14, 1–30.

Ennew, J. (1986) *The Sexual Exploitation of Children*. Cambridge: Polity Press.

Erlenmeyer-Kimling, L., Cornblatt, B.A., Bassett, A.S., Moldin, S.O., Hilldoff-Adamo, U. and Roberts, S. (1990) High-risk children in adolescence and young adulthood: course of global adjustment, in L.N. Robins and M. Rutter (eds) *Straight and Devious Pathways from Childhood to Adulthood*. Cambridge: Cambridge University Press.

Eth, S. and Pynoos, R.S. (1994) Children who witness the homicide of a parent, *Psychiatry: Interpersonal and Biological Processes*, 57(4): 287–306.

Ewalt, P.L. and Perkins, L. (1979) The real experience of death among adolescents: an empirical study, *Social Casework*, 60(9): 547–51.

Exley, C. and Letherby, G. (2001) Managing a disrupted lifecourse: issues of identity and emotion work, *Health*, 5(1): 112–32.

Eyetsemitan, F. (1998) Stifled grief in the workplace, *Death Studies*, 22(5): 469–79.

Farrington, D.P. (1996) *Understanding and Preventing Youth Crime: Social Policy Research 93*. York: Joseph Rowntree Foundation.

Featherstone, M. (1995) *The Body: Social Processes and Cultural Theory*. London: Sage.

Field, D. (1996) Awareness and modern dying, *Mortality*, 1(3): 255–66.

Field, D., Hockey, J. and Small, N. (1997) Making sense of difference: death, gender and ethnicity in modern Britain, in D. Field, J. Hockey and N. Small (eds) *Death, Gender and Ethnicity*. London: Routledge.

Finlay, I.G. and Jones, N.K. (2000) Unresolved grief in young offenders in prison, *British Journal of General Practice*, 50(456): 569–70.

Fleming, S.J. and Adolph, R. (1986) Helping bereaved adolescents: needs and responses, in C.A. Corr and J.N. McNeil (eds) *Adolescence and Death.* New York: Springer.

Fleming, S. and Balmer, L. (1996) Bereavement in adolescence, in C.A. Corr and D.E. Balk (eds) *Handbook of Adolescent Death and Bereavement.* New York: Springer.

Frantz, T.T., Farrell, M.M. and Trolley, B.C. (2001) Positive outcomes of losing a loved one, in R.A. Neimeyer (ed.) *Meaning Reconstruction and the Experience of Loss.* Washington, DC: American Psychological Association.

Fry, V. L. (2000) 'Part of me died too: creative strategies for grieving children and adolescents', in K.J. Doka (ed.) *Living with Grief: Children, Adolescents and Loss.* Brunner/Mazel/Hospice Foundation of America.

Furlong, A. and Cartmel, F. (1997) *Young People and Social Change: Individualization and Risk in Late Modernity.* Buckingham: Open University Press.

Garmezy, N. (1994) Reflections and commentary on risk, resilience, and development, in R.J. Haggerty, L.R. Sherrod, N. Garmezy and M. Rutter (eds) *Sress, Risk and Resilience in Children and Adolescents: Processes, Mechanisms, and Interventions.* Cambridge: Cambridge University Press.

Gerard, J.M. and Buehler, C. (2004) Cumulative environmental risk and youth maladjustment: the role of youth attributes, *Child Development,* 75(6): 1832–49.

Gersten, J.C., Beals, J. and Kallgren, C.A. (1991) Epidemiology and preventive interventions: parental death in childhood as an example, *American Journal of Community Psychiatry,* 19: 481–98.

Giddens, A. (1990) *The Consequences of Modernity.* Cambridge: Polity Press.

Giddens, A. (1991) *Modernity and Self Identity: Self and Society in the Late Modern Age.* Cambridge: Polity Press.

Giddens, A. (1992) *The Transformation of Intimacy: Sexuality, Love and Eroticism in Modern Societies.* Cambridge: Polity Press.

Giddens, A. (1999) *Runaway World: How Globalisation is Reshaping Our Lives.* London: Profile.

Gillies, J. and Neimeyer, R. (2006) Loss, grief and the search for significance: toward a model of meaning reconstruction in bereavement, *Journal of Constructivist Psychology,* 19(1): 31–65.

Gillies, V. (2001) Young people and family life: analysing and comparing disciplinary discourses, *Journal of Youth Studies,* 3(2): 211–28.

Gillies, V., Ribbens McCarthy, J. and Holland, J. (2001) *'Pulling Together: Pulling Apart': The Family Lives of Young People Aged 16–18.* London: Joseph Rowntree Foundation/Family Policy Studies Centre.

Gisborne, T. (1995) Death and bereavement in school: are you prepared? *Education,* June: 39–44.

Goffman, E. (1956) Embarrassment and social organisation, *American Journal of Sociology,* 62: 264–74.

Goleman, D. (1995) *Emotional Intelligence.* New York: Bantam.

Gordon, T. (2001) *A Need for Living: Signposts on the Journey of Life and Beyond.* Glasgow: Wild Goose Publications.

Gorer, G. (1987) *Death, Grief and Mourning in Contemporary Britain.* London: The Cresset Press.

Grant, L. and Schakner, B. (1993) Coping with the ultimate tragedy – the death of a student', *NASSP Bulletin* (April).

Gray, R.E. (1987) Adolescent response to the death of a parent, *Journal of Youth and Adolescence*, 16: 511–25.

Gray, R.E. (1989) Adolescents' perceptions of social support after the death of a parent, *Journal of Psychosocial Oncology*, 7: 127–44.

Griffiths, M. (2003) Terms of engagement – reaching hard to reach adolescents, *YoungMinds Magazine*, 62.

Grollman, E.A. (2000) To everything there is a season: empowering families and natural support systems, in K.J. Doka (ed.) *Living with Grief: Children, Adolescents and Loss*: Brunner/Mazel, Hospice Foundation of America.

Guerriero, A.M. and Fleming, S.J. (1985) Adolescent bereavement: a longitudinal study. Paper presented at the annual meeting of the Canadian Pscyhological Association, Halifax, Nova Scotia.

Gunaratnam, Y. (1997) Culture is not enough: a critique of multi-culturalism in palliative care, in D. Field, J. Hockey and N. Small (eds) *Death, Gender and Ethnicity*. London: Routledge.

Haggerty, R.J. (1994) *Stress, Risk and Resilience in Children and Adolescents: Processes, Mechanisms and Interventions.* Cambridge: Cambridge University Press.

Haine, R. A., Wolchick, S.A., Sander, I.N., Millsap, R.E. and Ayers, T.S. (2006) Positive parenting as a protective resource for parentally bereaved children, *Death Studies*, 30: 1–28.

Handsley, S. (2001) 'But what about us?' The residual effects of sudden death on self-identity and family relationships, *Mortality*, 6(1): 9–29.

Harrington, R. and Harrison, L. (1999) Unproven assumptions about the impact of bereavement on children, *Journal of the Royal Society of Medicine*, 92(5): 230–3.

Harrison, L. and Harrington, R. (2001) Adolescents' bereavement experiences: prevalence, association with depressive symptoms, and use of services, *Journal of Adolescence*, 24(2): 159–69.

Harrison, R. (2001) *Ordinary Days and Shattered Lives: Sudden Death and the Impact on Children and Families.* Buckinghamshire: The Child Bereavement Trust.

Hetherington, E. M. (ed.) (1999) *Coping with Divorce, Single Parenting and Remarriage.* Mahwah, NJ: Lawrence Erlbaum Associates.

Hetherington, E. M. (2003) Social support and the adjustment of children in divorced and remarried families, *Childhood: A Global Journal of Child Research*, 10(2): 217–53.

Higgins, S. (1999) Death education in the primary school, *International Journal of Children's Spirituality*, 4(1).

Hill, M. (1999) What's the problem? Who can help? The perspectives of children and young people on their well-being and on helping professionals, *Journal of Social Work Practice*, 13(2): 135–45.

Hockey, J. (1990) *Experiences of Death: An Anthropological Account*. Edinburgh: Edinburgh University Press.

Hogan, N. and DeSantis, L. (1994) Things that help and hinder adolescent sibling bereavement, *Western Journal of Nursing Research*, 16(2).

Holland, Janet (2002) Personal communication.

Holland, John (1993) Child bereavement in Humberside primary schools: short report, *Educational Research*, 35(3): 289–97.

Holland, John (2001) *Understanding Children's Experiences of Parental Bereavement*. London: Jessica Kingsley.

Holland, John (2004) Lost for Words in Hull, *Pastoral Care*, 22(4): 22–6.

Holland, John and Ludford, C. (1995) The effects of bereavement on children in Humberside secondary schools, *British Journal of Special Education*, 22(2): 56–9.

Holliday, J. (2002) *A Review of Sibling Bereavement – Impact and Interventions*. London: Barnardo's.

House of Commons Select Committee on Health (2004) *Palliative Care Fourth Report* on session 2003–4. London: House of Commons.

Ironside, V. (1996) *'You'll Get Over It': The Rage of Bereavement*. London: Penguin.

Jackson, M. and Colwell, J. (2001) Talking to children about death, *Mortality*, 6(3): 321–5.

James, A., Jenks, C. and Prout, A. (eds) (1998) *Theorizing Childhood*. Cambridge: Polity Press.

Janoff-Bulman, R. (1992) *Shattered Assumptions: Towards a Psychology of Trauma*. New York: The Free Press.

Job, N. and Frances, G. (2004) *Childhood Bereavement: Developing the Curriculum and Pastoral Support*. London: National Children's Bureau.

Johnson, C. (2002) Adolescent grief support groups, in D.W. Adams and E.J. Deveau (eds) *Beyond the Innocence of Childhood: Helping Children and Adolescents Cope with Death and Bereavement*, vol. 3. Amityville, NY: Baywood.

Johnston, L., MacDonald, R., Mason, P., Ridley, L. and Webster, C. (2000) *Snakes and Ladders: Young People, Transitions and Social Exclusion*. Bristol: Joseph Rowntree Foundation/Policy Press.

Jones, G. (2002) *The Youth Divide: Diverging Paths to Adulthood*. York: Joseph Rowntree Foundation.

Jones, G. (2005) *Young Adults and the Extension of Economic Dependence*. London: National Family and Parenting Institute.

Jonker, G. (1997) The many facets of Islam: death, dying and disposal between orthodox rule and historical convention, in C.M. Parkes, P. Laungani and B. Young (eds) *Death and Bereavement Across Cultures*. London: Routledge.

Katz, J. (2001) Supporting bereaved children at school, in J. Hockey, J. Katz and N.

Small (eds) *Grief, Mourning and Death Ritual*. Buckingham: Open University Press.

Kelle, U. (2005) Mixed methods as a means to overcome methodological limitations of qualitative and quantitative research. Paper presented at the ESRC-conference, *Mixed-methods: Identifying the Issues*, University of Manchester, October 26–8.

Kelly, J. (2003) Changing perspectives on children's adjustment following divorce: a view from the United States, *Childhood: A Global Journal of Child Research*, 10(3): 237–54.

Kenny, C. (1998) *A Thanatology of the Child: Children and Young People's Perceptions, Experiences and Understandings of Life, Death and Bereavement*. Dinton: Quay Books.

Kessler, R.C., Davis, C.G. and Kendler, K.S. (1997) Childhood adversity and adult psychiatric disorder in the US National Comorbidity Survey, *Psychological Medicine*, 27(5): 1101–19.

Kiernan, K. E. (1992) The impact of family disruption in childhood and transitions made in young adult life, *Population Studies*, 51: 213–34.

Kissane, D.W. and Bloch, S. (2002) *Family-focused Grief Therapy: A Model of Family-centred Care During Palliative Care and Bereavement*. Buckingham: Open University Press.

Klass, D., Silverman, P.R. and Nickman, S.L. (eds) (1996) *Continuing Bonds: New Understandings of Grief*. London: Taylor & Francis.

Kleinman, A. (1988) *The Illness Narratives: Suffering, Healing and the Human Condition*. New York: Basic Books.

Krementz, J. (1983) *How It Feels When a Parent Dies*, London: Victor Gollancz.

Kubler Ross, E. (1969) *On Death and Dying*. New York: Macmillan.

Kubler-Ross, E. (1981) *Living with Death and Dying*. London: Macmillan.

Leeds Animation Workshop (2002) *Grief in the Family*, narrated by Michael Rosen. Leeds: Leeds Animation Workshop.

Levete, S. (1998) *When People Die*. Brookfield, CT: Copper Beech Books.

Lewis, G. (2002) Introduction: expanding the social policy imaginary, in G. Lewis, S. Gewirtz and J. Clarke (eds) *Rethinking Social Policy*. London: Sage.

Liddle, M. and Solanki, A-R. (2002) *Persistent Young Offenders: Research on Individual Backgrounds and Life Experiences*. London: National Association for the Care and Resettlement of Offenders.

Lloyd-Williams, M. (1999) Rapid response, *British Medical Journal*, http://bmj.bmjjournals.com.libezproxy.open.ac.uk/cgi/eletters/319/7206/354.

Lloyd-Williams, M., Wilkinson, C. and Lloyd-Williams, F. (1998) Do bereaved children consult the primary health care team more frequently? *European Journal of Cancer Care*, 7: 120–4.

Loeber, R. and Dishion, T. (1983) Early predictors of male delinquency: a review, *Psychological Bulletin*, 94(1): 68–99.

Lowton, K. and Higginson, U. (2002) *Early Bereavement: What Factors Influence*

Children's Responses to Death. London: King's College London/National Council for Hospice and Specialist Palliative Care Services.

Luthar, S.S., Cicchetti, D. and Becker, B. (2000) The construct of resilience: a critical evaluation and guidelines for future work, *Child Development*, 71(3): 543–62.

Lutzke, J.R., Ayers, T.S., Sandler, I.N. and Barr, A. (1997) Risks and interventions for the parentally bereaved child, in S.A. Wolchik and I.N. Sandler (eds) *Handbook of Children's Coping: Linking Theory and Intervention*. New York: Plenum Press.

MacDonald, R. and Marsh, J. (2001) Disconnected youth? *Journal of Youth Studies*, 4(4): 373–93.

Machin, L. (1993) *Working with Young People in Loss Situations*. Harlow: Longman.

Mack, K.Y. (2001) Childhood family disruptions and adult well-being: the differential effects of divorce and parental death, *Death Studies*, 25(5): 419–43.

Mackay, N. (2003) Psychotherapy and the idea of meaning, *Theory and Psychology*, 13(3): 359–86.

Maclean, M. and Wadsworth, M.E.J. (1988) The interests of children after parental divorce: a long-term perspective, *International Journal of Law and the Family*, 2: 155–66.

Maclean, M. and Kuh, D. (1991) The long-term effects for girls of parental divorce, in M. Maclean and D. Groves (eds) *Women's Issues in Social Policy*. London: Routledge.

Mallon, B. (1998) *Helping Children to Manage Loss: Positive Strategies for Renewal and Growth*. London: Jessica Kingsley.

Marris, P. (1996) *The Politics of Uncertainty: Attachment in Private and Public Life*. London: Routledge.

Martinson, I.M. and Campos, R. D. (1991) Adolescent bereavement: long-term responses to a sibling death from cancer, *Journal of Adolescent Research*, 6: 54–69.

Martinson, I.M., Davies, E. B. and McClowry, S.G. (1987) The long-term effects of sibling death on self-concept, *Journal of Pediatric Nursing*, 2: 227–35.

Masson, J. and Gieve, K. (2003) Discussion of paper presented by Judith Aldridge, 'Medical Practice and New Thinking About Children', *Frameworks of Understanding: Multidisciplinary Perspectives on Childhood*. Leeds: Leeds University.

Maybin, J. and Woodhead, M. (eds) (2003) *Childhoods in Context*. Chichester: Wiley in association with the Open University.

McBride, J. and Simms, S. (2001) Death in the family: adapting a family systems framework to the grief process, *American Journal of Family Therapy*, 29(1): 59–73.

McCord, J. (1982) A longitundinal view of the relationship between paternal absence and crime, in J. Gunn and D.P. Farrington (eds) *Abnormal Offenders, Delinquency and the Criminal Justice System*, Vol. 1. Chichester: Wiley.

McCord, J. (1990) Long-term perspectives on parental absence, in L.N. Robins and

M. Rutter (eds) *Straight and Devious Pathways from Childhood to Adulthood.* Cambridge: Cambridge University Press.

McNally, D. (2005) *The Influence of Social Contexts on Bereavement: A Qualitative Study of Adults Bereaved During Childhood and Adolescence Due to the Northern Ireland Troubles.* Unpublished dissertation, MSc in Social Research Methods, Open University.

Mellor, P. (1993) *The Sociology of Death.* Oxford: Blackwell.

Meltzer, H. and Gatward, R., with Goodman, R. and Ford, T. (2000) *The Mental Health of Children and Adolescents in Great Britain: The Report of a Survey Carried out in 1999 by Social Survey Division of the Office for National Statistics on behalf of the Department of Health, the Scottish Health Executive and the National Assembly for Wales.* London: The Stationery Office.

Miller, S. (1997) *After Death: How People Around the World Map the Journey After Life.* New York: Simon & Schuster.

Mireault, G. and Bond, A. L. (1992) Parental death in childhood: perceived vulnerability, and adult depression and anxiety, *American Journal of Orthopsychiatry* 62(4): 517–24.

Mireault, G., Bearor, K. and Thomas, T. (2001) Adult romantic attachment among women who experienced childhood maternal loss, *Omega Journal of Death and Dying*, 44(1): 97–104.

Mitchell, R., Dorling, D. and Shaw, M. (2000) *Inequalities in Life and Death: What if Britain were More Equal?* Bristol: Policy Press/Joseph Rowntree Foundation.

Monroe, B. (1995) It is impossible NOT to communicate – helping the bereaved family, in S.C. Smith and M. Pennells (eds) *Interventions with Bereaved Children.* London: Jessica Kingsley.

Monroe, B. and Kraus, F. (eds) (2005) *Brief Interventions with Bereaved Children.* Oxford: Oxford University Press.

Moran, J. (2002) *Interdisciplinarity.* London: Routledge.

Morgan, D. and Wilkinson, I. (2001) The problem of suffering and the sociological task of theodicy, *Europen Journal of Social Theory*, 4(2): 199–214.

Morgan, J.D. (2002) Some concluding observations, in J.D. Morgan and P. Laungani (eds) *Death and Bereavement Around the World. Volume 1: Major Religious Traditions.* Amytiville, NY: Baywood.

Morin, S.M. and Welsh, L.A. (1996) Adolescents' perceptions and experiences of death and grieving, *Adolescence*, 31(123): 585–95.

Moss, B. (2002) *Spirituality: A Personal View.* Basingstoke: Palgrave.

Muir Gray, J.A. (2001) *Evidence-Based Healthcare*, 2nd edn. Edinburgh: Churchill Livingstone.

Murphy, P.A. (1986) Parental death in childhood and loneliness in young adults, *Omega Journal of Death and Dying*, 17(3): 219–28.

Murray, J.A. (2001) Loss as a universal concept: a review of the literature to identify common aspects of loss in diverse situations. *Journal of Loss and Trauma*, 6(3): 219–241.

Nadeau, J.W. (1990) *Families Making Sense of Death*. London: Sage.

Nadeau, J.W. (2002) Family construction of meaning, in R.A. Neimeyer (ed.) *Meaning Reconstruction and the Experience of Loss*. Washington, DC: American Psychological Association.

National Children's Bureau (2003) *Factsheet on PSHE/Citizenship Education*. London: National Children's Bureau.

Nazroo, J.Y. (2001) *Ethnicity, Class and Health*. London: Policy Studies Institute.

Neimeyer, R.A. (2000) Searching for the meaning of meaning: grief therapy and the process of reconstruction, *Death Studies*, 24(6): 541–58.

Neimeyer, R. A. (ed.) (2001) *Meaning Reconstruction and the Experience of Loss*. Washington: American Psychological Association.

Neimeyer, R. A. (2002) Making sense of loss, in K.J. Doka (ed.) *Living with Grief: Loss in Later Life*. Washington, DC: Hospice Foundation of America.

Neimeyer, R.A. and Anderson, A. (2002) Meaning reconstruction theory, in N. Thompson (ed.) *Loss and Grief: A Guide for Human Service Practitioners*. Basingstoke: Palgrave.

Neimeyer, R.A. and Hogan, N. (2001) Quantitative or qualitative? Measurement issues in the study of grief, in M.S. Stroebe, R.O. Hansson, W. Stroebe and H. Schut (eds) *Handbook of Bereavement Research*. Washington, DC: American Psychological Association.

Neimeyer, R.A., Prigerson, H., Holly G. and Davies, B. (2002) Mourning and meaning, *American Behavioral Scientist*, 46(2): 235–51.

Neuberger, J. (1987) *Caring for Dying People of Different Faiths*. London: Austen Cornish Publishers.

Newburn, T. and Shiner, M. (2001) *Teenage Kicks: Young People and Alcohol – A Review of the Literature*. York: Joseph Rowntree Foundation.

Newman, T. (2002) *Promoting Resilience: A Review of Effective Strategies for Child Care Services*. Exeter: University of Exeter.

Norwich, J. of (1998) *Revelations of Divine Love*. London: Penguin.

O'Brien, J. Goodenow, C. Espin, O. (1991) Adolescents' reactions to the death of a peer, *Adolescence*, 26(102): 431–40.

O'Hara, D.M., Taylor, R. and Simpson, K. (1994) Critical incident stress de-briefing: bereavement support in schools – developing a role for an LEA educational psychology service, *Educational Psychology in Practice*, 10(1): 27–34.

Oswin, M. (1991) *'Am I Allowed to Cry?' A Study of Bereavement Amongst People who have Learning Difficulties*. London: Souvenir Press.

Papadatou, D., Metallinou, O., Hatzichristou, C. and Pavlidi, L. (2002) Supporting the bereaved child: teachers' perceptions and experiences in Greece, *Mortality*, 7(3): 324–39.

Parke, J. (1999) Emotional literacy: education for meaning, *International Journal of Children's Spirtuality*, 4(1): 19–28.

Parkes, C.M. (1998) *Bereavement*. Harmondsworth: Penguin.

Parkes, C. M. (2005) Grief and bereavement in Contemporary society: reflections on current thinking, Paper presented at the 7th International Conference on Grief and Bereavement in Contemporary Society, King's College, London.

Parkes, C.M., Laungani, P. and Young, B. (1997) Introduction, in C.M. Parkes, P. Laungani and B. Young (eds) *Death and Bereavement Across Cultures*. London: Routledge.

Patterson, G.R., DeBaryshe, B.D. and Ramsey, E. (1989) A developmental perspective on antisocial behaviour, *American Psychologist*, 44(2): 329–35.

Pennells, M. and Smith, S.C. (1995) *The Forgotten Mourners: Guidelines for Working with Bereaved Children*. London: Jessica Kingsley.

Perschy, M.K. (1997) *Helping Teens Work Through Grief*. Washington, DC: Accelerated Development.

Pfeffer, C. R., Karus, D., Siegel, K. and Jiang, H. (2000) Child survivors of parental death from cancer or suicide: depressive and behavioral outcomes, *Psycho-Oncology*, 9(1): 1–10.

Pfeffer, C.R., Jiang, H., Kakuma, T., Hwang, J. and Metsch, M. (2002) Group intervention for children bereaved by the suicide of a relative, *Journal of the American Academy of Child and Adolescent Psychiatry*, 41(5): 505–13.

Pfefferbaum, B., Nixon, S.J., Tucker, P.M., Tivis, R.D., Moore, V.L., Gurwitch, R. H., Pynoos, R.S. and Geis, H.K. (1999) Posttraumatic stress responses in bereaved children after the Oklahoma City bombing, *Journal of the American Academy of Child and Adolescent Psychiatry*, 38(11): 1372–9.

Pietila, M. (2002) Support groups: a psychological or social device for suicide bereavement? *British Journal of Guidance and Counselling*, 30(4): 401–14.

Prigerson, H. (2005) Research to validate diagnostic criteria for complicated grief, Paper presented at the 7th International Conference on Grief and Bereavement in Contemporary Society, King's College London.

Raphael, B. (1984) *The Anatomy of Bereavement: A Handbook for the Caring Professionals*. London: Unwin Hyman.

Rask, K., Kaunonen, M. and Paunonen-Ilmonen, M. (2002) Adolescent coping with grief after the death of a loved one, *International Journal of Nursing Practice*, 8: 137–42.

Raskin, J.D. and Neimeyer, R.A. (2003) Coherent constructivism: a response to Mackay, *Theory and Psychology*, 13(3): 397–402.

Raviv, A., Sadeh, A., Silberstein, O. and Diver, O. (2000) Young Israelis' reactions to national trauma: the Rabin assassination and terror attacks, *Political Psychology*, 21(2): 299–322.

Reid, J. (2002) School management and eco-system support for bereaved children and their teachers, *International Journal of Children's Spirituality*, 7(2): 193–207.

Reinherz, H.Z., Giaconia, R.M., Pakiz, B., Silverman, A.B., Frost, A.K. and Lefkowitz, E.S. (1993) Psychosocial risks for major depression in late adolescence – a longitudinal community study, *Journal of the American Academy of Child and Adolescent Psychiatry*, 32(6): 1155–63.

Reinherz, H. Z. *et al.* (1999) Major depression in the transition to adulthood: risks and impairments, *Journal of Abnormal Psychology*, 108(3): 500–10.

Renn, P. (2000) The link between childhood trauma and later violent offending: a case study, in G. Boswell (ed.) *Violent Children and Adolescents: Asking the Question Why?* London: Whurr.

Rheingold, A.A., Smith D.W., Ruggerio, K.J., Saunders, B.E., Kilpatrick, D.G., Resnick, H.S. (2004) Loss, trauma exposure and mental health in a representative sample of 12–17-year-old youth: data from the national survey of adolscents, *Journal of Loss and Trauma* January–March, 9(1): 1–19.

Ribbens, J. (1994) *Mothers and their Children: A Sociology of Childrearing*. London: Sage.

Ribbens, J. and Edwards, R. (eds) (1998) *Feminist Dilemmas in Qualitative Research: Public Knowledge and Private Lives*. London: Sage.

Ribbens McCarthy, J. (forthcoming) Re-presenting academic knowledge: power and responsibility in the processes of doing a literature review, in V. Gillies and H. Lucey (eds) *Power, Knowledge and the Academy: Exploring the Institutional and Personal Dynamics of Research*. London: Sage.

Ribbens McCarthy, J. and Edwards, R. (2000) Moral tales of the child and the adult: narratives of contemporary family lives under changing circumstances, *Sociology*, 34(4): 785–804.

Ribbens McCarthy, J. and Edwards, R. (2002) The individual in public and private: the significance of mothers and children, in A. Carling, S. Duncan and R. Edwards (eds) *Analysing Families: Morality and Rationality in Policy and Practice*. London: Routledge.

Ribbens McCarthy, J. and Jessop, J. (2005) *Young People, Bereavement and Loss: Disruptive Transitions?* London: Joseph Rowntree Foundation/National Children's Bureau.

Riches, G. (2002) Gender and sexism, in N. Thompson (ed.) *Loss and Grief: A Guide for Human Services Practitioners*. Basingstoke: Palgrave.

Riches, G. and Dawson, P. (2000) *An Intimate Loneliness: Supporting Bereaved Parents and Siblings*. Buckingham: Open University Press.

Rickgarn, R.L.V. (1996) The need for postvention on college campuses: a rationale and case study findings, in C.A. Corr and D.E. Balk (eds) *Handbook of Adolescent Death and Bereavement*. New York: Springer.

Rigazio-DiGilio, S.A. (2001) Videography: re-storying the lives of clients facing terminal illness, in R. Neimeyer (ed.) *Meaning Reconstruction and the Experience of Loss*. Cambridge: Cambridge University Press.

Ringler, L.L. and Hayden, D.C. (2000) Adolescent bereavement and social support: peer loss compared to other losses, *Journal of Adolescent Research*, 15(2): 209–30.

Robins, L.N. and Rutter, M. (eds) (1990) *Straight and Devious Pathways from Childhood to Adulthood*. Cambridge: Cambridge University Press.

Rodgers, B. (1990) Adult affective disorder and early environment, *British Journal of Psychiatry*, 157: 539–50.

Rodgers, B. and Pryor, J. (1998) *Divorce and Separation: The Outcomes for Children*. York: Joseph Rowntree Foundation.

Roeser, R. W., van der Wolf, K. and Strobel, K.R. (2001) On the relation between social-emotional and school functioning during early adolescence – preliminary findings from Dutch and American samples, *Journal of School Psychology*, 39(2): 111–39.

Rolls, L. and Payne, S. (2003) Childhood bereavement services: a survey of UK provision, *Palliative Medicine*, 17: 423–32.

Rose, N. (1989) *Governing the Soul: The Shaping of the Private Self*. London: Routledge.

Rosenblatt, P.C. (2001) A social constructionist perspective on cultural differences in grief, in M. Stroebe, W. Stroebe, R. Hansson and H. Schut (eds) *Handbook of Bereavement Research: Consequences, Coping, Care*. Washington, DC: American Psychological Association.

Rowling, L. (1995) The disenfranchised grief of teachers, *Omega Journal of Death and Dying*, 31(4): 317–29.

Rowling, L. (2003) *Grief in School Communities: Effective Support Strategies*. Buckingham: Open University Press.

Rowling, L. and Holland, J. (2000) Grief and school communities: the impact of social context, a comparison between Australia and England, *Death Studies*, 24(1): 35–50.

Rubel, B. (2005) Identifying ways school nurses can support grieving children and adolescents, *School Nurse News*, 22(1): 29–34.

Rutter, M. (2000) Psychosocial influences: critiques, findings and research needs, *Development and Psychopathology*, 12(3): 375–405.

Rutter, M., Giller, H. and Hagell, A. (1998) *Anti-Social Behaviour by Young People*. Cambridge: Cambridge University Press.

Saldinger, A., Poerterfield, K., and Cain, A.C. (2004) 'Meeting the needs of parentally bereaved, children: a framework for child-centered parenting'. *Psychiatry* Winter 67(4): 331–52.

Saler, L. and Skolnick, N. (1992) Childhood parental death and depression in adulthood – roles of surviving parent and family environment, *American Journal of Orthopsychiatry*, 62(4): 504–16.

Salloum, A., Avery, L. and McClain, R.P. (2001) Group psychotherapy for adolescent survivors of homicide victims: a pilot study, *Journal of the American Academy of Child and Adolescent Psychiatry*, 40(11): 1261–7.

Salter, A. and Stubbs, D. (2004) Feeling alone … getting help from the internet, Paper presented at the Childhood Bereavement Network Conference, Feeling Alone and Different. London 28th April.

Saltzman, W.R., Pynoos, R.S., Layne, C.M., Steinberg, A.M. and Aisenberg, E. (2001) Trauma- and grief-focused intervention for adolescents exposed to community violence: results of a school-based screening and group treatment protocol, *Group Dynamics: Theory Research and Practice*, 5(4): 291–303.

Sandler, I. N. Wolchik, S.A., Mackinnon, D., Ayers, T.S. and Roosa, M.W. (1997) Developing linkages between theory and intervention in stress and coping processes, in S.A. Wolchik and I.N. Sandler (eds) *Handbook of Children's Coping: Linking Theory and Intervention*. New York: Plenum Press.

Sandler, I. N. *et al.* (2003) The Family Bereavement Program: efficacy evaluation of a theory-based prevention program for parentally bereaved children and adolescents, *Journal of Consulting and Clinical Psychology*, 71(3): 587–600.

Schachter, S. (1992) Adolescent experiences with the death of a peer, *Omega Journal of Death and Dying*, 24(1): 1–11.

Scheper-Hughes, N. (1992) *Death Without Weeping: The Violence of Everyday Life in Brazil*. Berkeley, CA: California University Press.

Schneiderman, G. (1993) Adolescent mourning after the accidental death of a peer,' *Humane Medicine*, 9(3): 216–19.

Schneiderman, G., Winders, R.N., Tallett, S. and Feldman, W. (1994) Do child and parent bereavement programs work? *Canadian Journal of Psychiatry*, 39: 215–17.

Schoon, I. and Montgomery, S. M. (1997) The relationship between early life experiences and adult depression, *Zeitschrift Fur Pscyhosomatiische Medizin Und Psychoanalyse*, 43(4): 319–33.

Schoon, I. and Parsons, S. (2002) Competence in the face of adversity: the impact of early family environment and long-term consequences, *Children and Society*, 16: 260–72.

Schuman, J. (1998) Childhood, infant and perinatal mortality, 1996: social and biological factors in deaths of children aged under 3, *Population Trends*, 92(Summer): 5–16.

Schut, H. (2005) Balancing research and counselling: on the need for reciprocity in understanding grief, Paper presented at the 7th International Conference on Grief and Bereavement in Contemporary Society, King's College, London.

Schut, H., Stroebe, M.S., van den Bout, J. and Terheggen, M. (2002) The efficacy of bereavement interventions: determining who benefits, in M.S. Stroebe, R.O. Hansson, W. Stroebe and H. Schut (eds) *Handbook of Bereavement Research: Consequences, Coping and Care*. Washington, DC: American Psychological Association.

Schutz, A. (1954) Concept and theory formation in the social sciences, *Journal of Philosophy*, 51: 257–73.

Seale, C. (1998) *Constructing Death. The Sociology of Dying and Bereavement*. Cambridge: Cambridge University Press.

Seale, C. (2001) An historical approach to medical knowledge, in C. Seale, S. Pattison and B. Davey (eds) *Medical Knowledge: Doubt and Certainty*, 2nd edn. Buckingham: Open University Press.

Seiffge-Krenke, I. (2000) Causal links between stressful events, coping style and adolescent symptomology, *Journal of Adolescence*, 23(6): 675–91.

Servaty, H.L. and Hayslip, B. (2001) Adjustment to loss among adolescents, *Omega Journal of Death and Dying*, 43(4): 311–30.

Sharp, P. (2000) Promoting emotional literacy: emotional literacy improves and increases your life chances, *Pastoral Care*, 18(3): 8–10.

Sharp, P. and Faupel, A. (eds) (2002) *Promoting Educational Literacy: Guidelines for Schools, Local Authorities and the Health Services*. Southampton: Emotional Literacy Group, Southampton City Council Local Education Authority.

Sharp, S. and Cowie, H. (1998) *Counselling and Supporting Children in Distress*. London: Sage.

Shaw, M. (1999) *The Widening Gap* Bristol: Policy Press.

Shears, J. (1995) Managing tragedy in a secondary school, in S.C. Smith and M. Pennells (eds) *Interventions with Bereaved Children*. London: Jessica Kingsley.

Sheras, P.L. (2000) *Grief and Traumatic Loss: What Schools Need to Know and Do*. Washington, DC: Hospice Foundation of America.

Shoebridge, P. and Gowers, S. G. (2000) Parental high concern and adolescent-onset anorexia nervosa – A case-control study to investigate direction of causality, *British Journal of Psychiatry*, 176: 132–7.

Shoor, M. and Speed, M. (1963) Death, delinquency and the mourning process, in R. Fulton (ed.) *Death and Identity*. Barie, MD: Charles Press.

Silverman, P.R. (2000) *Never too Young to Know: Death in Children's Lives*. New York: Oxford University Press.

Silverman, P.R. and Worden, J.W. (1992) Children's reactions in the early months after the death of a parent, *American Journal of Orthopsychiatry*, 62: 93–503.

Small, N. (2001) Theories of grief: a critical review, in J. Hockey, J. Katz and N. Small (eds) *Grief, Mourning and Death Ritual*. Buckingham: Open University Press.

Small, N. and Hockey, J. (2001) *Discourse into Practice: The Production of Bereavement Care*. Buckingham: Open University Press.

Small, S. and Memmo, M. (2004) Contemporary models of youth development and problem prevention: toward an integration of terms, concepts and models, *Family Relations*, 53(1): 3–11.

Smart, C. (2003) Introduction: new perspectives on childhood and divorce, *Childhood: A Global Journal of Child Research*, 10(2): 123–30.

Smith, S. and Browne, J. (2004) Feeling alone . . . at the hospital, Paper presented to the Childhood Bereavement Network Conference, Feeling Alone and Different. London: 28th April.

Smith, S.C. and Pennells, M. (eds) (1995) *Interventions with Bereaved Children*. London: Jessica Kingsley.

Sorensen, J.R. (1989) Responding to student or teacher death: preplanning crisis intervention, *Journal of Counseling and Development*, 67: 426–7.

Spall, B. and Jordan, G. (1999) Teachers' perspectives on working with children experiencing loss, *Pastoral Care*, 17(3): 3–7.

Stevenson, R.G. (2000) *The Role of Death Education in Helping Children to Cope with Loss*. Washington, DC: Hospice Foundation of America.

Stokes, J. (2004) *Then, Now and Always: Supporting Children as They Journey Through Grief: A Guide for Practitioners*. Cheltenham: Winston's Wish.

Stokes, J., Wyver, S. and Crossley, D. (1997) The challenge of evaluating a bereavement programme, *Palliative Medicine*, 11: 179–90.

Stokes, J., Pennington, J., Monroe, B., Papadatou, D. and Relf, M. (1999) Developing services for bereaved children: a discussion of the theoretical and practical issues involved, *Mortality*, 4(3): 291–307.

Stone, B. (2004) Towards a writing without power: notes on the narration of madness, *Auto/biography*, 12(1): 16–33.

Strange, J.-M. (2005) *Death, Grief and Poverty in Britain, 1870–1914*. Cambridge: Cambridge University Press.

Strathern, M. (1992) *After Nature: English Kinship in the Late Twentieth Century*. Cambridge: Cambridge University Press.

Stroebe, M. and Schut, H. (1995) *The Dual Process Model of Coping with Loss*. Oxford: St Catherine's College.

Stroebe, M. and Schut, H. (1999) The dual process model of coping with bereavement: rationale and description, *Death Studies*, 23(3).

Stuber, J. *et al.* (2002) Determinants of counseling for children in Manhattan after the September 11 attacks, *Psychiatric Services*, 53(7): 815–22.

Sutcliffe, P., Tufnell, G. and Cornish, U. (eds) (1998) *Working with the Dying and Bereaved: Systemic Approaches to Therapeutic Work*. London: Macmillan.

Sweeting, H., West, P. and Richards, M.P.M. (1998) Teenage family life, lifestyles and life chances: associations with family structure, conflict with parents, and joint family activity, *International Journal of Law, Policy and the Family*, 12: 15–46.

Tedeschi, R.G. (1996) Support groups for bereaved adolescents, in C.A. Corr and D.E. Balk (eds) *Handbook of Adolescent Death and Bereavement*. New York: Springer.

Tennant, C., Bebbington, B. and Hurry, J. (1980) Parental death in childhood and risk of adult depressive disorders: a review, *Psychological Medicine*, 10: 289–99.

Thompson, M. P. *et al.* (1998) Psychological symptomatology following parental death in a predominantly minority sample of children and adolescents, *Journal of Clinical Child Psychology*, 27(4): 434–41.

Thompson, N. (ed.) (2002) *Loss and Grief: A Guide for Human Services Practitioners*. Basingstoke: Palgrave.

Thomson, R. *et al.* (2002) Critical moments: choice, chance and opportunity in young people's narratives of transition, *Sociology*, 36(2): 335–54.

Tremblay, G. and Israel, A. (1998) Children's adjustment to parental death, *Clinical Psychology*, 5: 424–38.

Tyson-Rawson, K.J. (1996) Adolescent response to the death of a parent, in C.A.

Corr and D.E. Balk (eds) *Handbook of Adolescent Death and Bereavement*. New York: Springer.

Van Eerdewegh, M.M., Bieri, M.D., Parrilla, R.H. and Clayton, P.J. (1982) The bereaved child, *British Journal of Psychiatry*, 140: 23–9.

Wadsworth, M.E.J. (1979) *Roots of Delinquency: Infancy, Adolescence and Crime*. Oxford: Martin Robertson.

Wadsworth, M. E. J. (1991) *The Imprint of Time: Childhood, History and Adult Life*. Oxford: Clarendon Press.

Wadsworth, M.E.J. and Maclean, M. (1986) Parents' divorce and children's later life chances, *Children and Youth Services Review*, 8: 145–59.

Wallbank, S. (1991) *Facing Grief: Bereavement and the Young Adult*. Cambridge: Lutterworth Press.

Walter, T. (1991) Modern death: taboo or not taboo? *Sociology*, 25(2): 293–310.

Walter, T. (1999) *On Bereavement: The Culture of Grief*. Buckingham: Open University Press.

Ward, B. (1996) *Good Grief: Exploring Feelings, Loss and Death with Under Elevens: A Holistic Approach*, 2nd edn. London: Jessica Kingsley.

Wass, H. (2004) A perspective on the current state of death education, *Death Studies*, 28(4): 289–308.

Weare, K. (2004) *Developing the Emotionally Literate School*. London: Sage.

Webb, N.B. (2000) Play therapy to help bereaved children, in K.J. Doka (ed.) *Living with Grief: Children, Adolescents and Loss*. Brunner/Mazel/Hospice Foundation of America.

Wells, L.E. and Rankin, J.H. (1991) Families and delinquency: a meta-analysis of the impact of broken homes, *Social Problems*, 38: 71–93.

West, D.J. and Farrington, D.P. (1973) *Who Becomes Delinquent?* London: Heinemann.

Wetherell, M., Taylor, S. and Yates, S.J. (eds) (2001) *Discourse Theory and Practice: A Reader*. London: Sage.

Wheeler, S.R. and Austin, J. (2000) The loss response list: a tool for measuring adolescent grief responses, *Death Studies*, 24(1): 21–34.

Wilby, J. (1995) Transcultural counselling: bereavement counselling with adolescents, in S.C. Smith and M. Pennells (eds) *Interventions with Bereaved Children*. London: Jessica Kingsley.

Wild, S. and Mckeigue, P. (1997) Cross-sectional analysis of mortality by country of birth in England and Wales 1970–92, *British Medical Journal*, 314(705).

Wilkinson, I. (2005) *Suffering: A Sociological Introduction*. Cambridge: Polity Press.

Wilson, A. *et al.* (2003) *Schools and Family Change: School Based Support for Children Experiencing Divorce and Separation*. York: Joseph Rowntree Foundation.

Winton, P. (2002) A personal perspective, *Childhood Bereavement Network Bulletin*, October: 3–4.

Wolfe, B.S. and Senta, L.M. (2002) Interventions with bereaved children nine to thirteen years of age: from a medical center based young person's grief support program, in D.W. Adams and E.J. Deveau (eds) *Beyond the Innocence of Childhood, Vol. 3, Helping Children and Adolescents Cope with Death and Bereavement.* New York: Baywood.

Wood, C. and Baulkwill, J. (1995) Sharing experiences – the value of groups for bereaved children, in S. C. Smith and M. Pennells (eds) *Interventions with Bereaved Children.* London: Jessica Kingsley.

Worden, J.W. (1996) *Children and Grief: When a Parent Dies.* New York: Guilford Press.

Worden, J.W., Davies, B. and McCown, D. (1999) Comparing parent loss with sibling loss, *Death Studies*, 23(1).

Wrenn, L. (1991) College student death: postvention issues for educators and counsellors, in D. Papadatou and C. Papadotos (eds) *Children and Death.* New York: Hemisphere.

Wright, B.J., Aldridge, J., Gillance, H. and Tucker, A. (1996) Hospice-based groups for bereaved siblings, *European Journal of Palliative Care*, 3(1): 10–15.

Wyn, J. and White, R. (1997) *Rethinking Youth.* London: Sage.

Young, B. and Papadatou, D. (1997) Childhood, death and bereavement across cultures, in C.M. Parkes, P. Laungani and B. Young (eds) *Death and Bereavement Across Cultures.* London: Routledge.

Youth Justice Trust (2001) *A Survey of Some of the General and Specific Health Issues for Youth Offending Teams.* Greater Manchester: Youth Justice Trust.

Youth Justice Trust (2003a) *Grief, Loss and Developing Resilience.* Manchester: Greater Manchester Youth Justice Trust.

Youth Justice Trust (2003b) *The Health of Children and Young People who are Involved with the Greater Manchester Youth Offending Teams (YOTs).* Manchester: Greater Manchester Youth Justice Trust.

Youth Justice Trust (2003c) *On the Case: A Survey of Over 1000 Children and Young People Under Supervision by Youth Offending Teams in Greater Manchester and West Yorkshire.* Manchester: Youth Justice Trust.

Zelizer, V.A. (1994) *Pricing the Priceless Child: The Changing Social Value of Children.* Princeton, NJ: Princeton University Press.

Index

GRIEF IN SCHOOL COMMUNITIES

Effective Support Strategies

Louise Rowling

This book is an essential guide for all members of a school community and other professionals who need to know how to be supportive in times of crisis – including social workers, psychologists and bereavement specialists. Whilst the emphasis of many books about young people and loss and grief has been on how to support those young people as individuals in a family context, this book takes a different approach and uses 'the school community' as the organizing supportive framework. This approach recognizes that losses are embedded in a young person's social environment – the school and its community, as well as the family. The theoretical orientation utilised is that death and all loss experiences are interpreted through social interaction and experienced within a social context.

The book is firmly based on theory, research and practice. It breaks new ground in demonstrating the components in a school that can be used to support grieving individuals in times of personal crisis and to support whole school communities when traumatic incidents occur. Within this comprehensive approach attention is given to the needs and experiences of personnel – teachers, students, school leaders, parents; as well as school policies and programs and links with outside services.

Contents
Foreword – Preface – Acknowledgements – Frameworks for a comprehensive approach to loss and grief in schools – Impact of loss on children and adolescents – Teachers being human – Grief and the classroom – Critical incident management – Supportive school environment – Being in charge – Grief and family/school relationships – Partnerships with outside agencies – Special cases – Disenfranchised grief in schools – Education and training – References – Index.

208pp 0 335 21115 1 (Paperback)   0 335 21116 X (Hardback)

FAMILY FOCUSED GRIEF THERAPY

David W. Kissane and Sidney Bloch

"To those of us who have been aware of the innovative service to families facing death and bereavement that has been developed by David W. Kissane and Sidney Bloch this book has been eagerly awaited. Their work is a logical development in the field of Palliative Care in which it has long been recognized that, when life is threatened, it is the family (which includes the patient) which is, or ought to be, the unit of care. The work also has great relevance for the wider field of bereavement care...all who work to help families at times of death and bereavement will find much to learn from this book which represents a useful addition to our understanding of the losses which, sooner or later, we all have to face." – Colin Murray Parkes

Family members are often intimately involved in the care of dying people and themselves require support through both their experience of palliative care and bereavement. This innovative book describes a comprehensive model of family care and how to go about it – *Family Focused Grief Therapy* is an approach which is new, preventive, cost effective and with proven benefits to bereaved people. It describes a highly original and creative approach to bereavement care, one likely to revolutionize psychosocial care in oncology, hospice or palliative care and grief work.

The book has been designed rather like a therapy manual, providing a step-by-step approach to assessment and intervention. Its rich illustration through many clinical examples brings the process of therapy alive for the reader, anticipating the common challenges that arise and describing how the therapist might respond. Families are recognised throughout as the central social unit, pivotal to the success of palliative care.

Family Focused Grief Therapy will be of use to doctors, nurses, psychologists, social workers, pastoral care workers, psychiatrists and other allied health professionals who work in caring for the dying and for their bereaved relatives. Based soundly on a decade of internationally regarded research, this book will alter the direction of future medical practice and is destined to become a classic in its field.

Contents

272pp 0 335 20349 3 (Paperback)   0 335 20350 7 (Hardback)

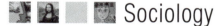
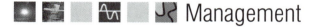
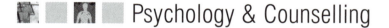
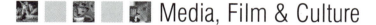
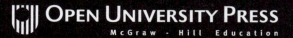
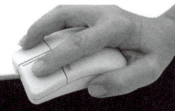